Finding
Sufficiency

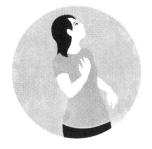

Breastfeeding With
Insufficient
Glandular Tissue

Diana Cassar-Uhl, MPH, IBCLC

Praeclarus Press, LLC
2504 Sweetgum Lane
Amarillo, Texas 79124 USA
806-367-9950
www.PraeclarusPress.com

DISCLAIMER
The information contained in this publication is advisory only and is not intended to replace sound clinical judgment or individualized patient care. The author disclaims all warranties, whether expressed or implied, including any warranty as the quality, accuracy, safety, or suitability of this information for any particular purpose.

ISBN: 978-1-9398071-2-0

Cover Design: Ken Tackett
Acquisition & Development: Kathleen Kendall-Tackett
Copy Editing: Janell E. Robisch, Kathleen Kendall-Tackett
Layout & Design: Cornelia Georgiana Murariu
Operations: Scott Sherwood

Table of Contents

Foreword

I became a mother in the "everyone can breastfeed if you only TRY hard enough" era. Even 13 years later, I encounter this kind of thinking almost daily. I call it an era because, while I believe that for many mothers, this belief still reigns supreme, my hope is that a tide is finally turning. We, as a culture, are waking up to the reality that for some women, effort will never be enough to meet their breastfeeding goals. But I also take hope in the flip-side...that when we recognize and understand the many nuances that are at play in our biologically driven ability to make milk, we will also embrace the truth that breastfeeding is about so much more than nutrition and sustenance. For the women who will read this book, and for the volunteers and professionals who will support them, I pray you find hope here.

I first met Diana Cassar-Uhl in the crowded basement of a trendy Manhattan salon. We were both attending a fundraising event sponsored by Best for Babes (www.bestforbabes.org) and my colleague, Monique Jones, and I had taken a bus from Washington, DC to attend. I was a brand-spanking-new International Board Certified Lactation Consultant (IBCLC), still very green around the edges and not quite believing I had met my goal of becoming a breastfeeding professional. Diana was one of the speakers for the evening. I was struck, quite quickly, by her approachable exper- tise. We struck up a conversation and it is one of those that I wish, years later, I had recorded. We immediately found a huge swath of common ground and quickly friended each other on Facebook, followed each other on Twitter, and exchanged numbers so we could continue our conversations by text (as typical of our culture's current communication norms!).

I'm not sure we've stopped talking since. Diana has not only become one of my dearest friends, but also my constant "go to" IBCLC when I feel out of my depth. Her ability to recall references and scientific studies is brilliant and almost before I finish my "What do you know about..." queries, she's sending on links to relevant research. We've attended countless conferences together, shared late-night musings about the state of lactation in the world, and engaged in constant texting where we talk about everything from nipple shields to mothering our delightfully quirky pre-teens. I've jokingly referred to her as my "Lactation BFF," but the truth is that her influence has made me an exceedingly better lactation consultant.

One of the things we share in common is a fierce commitment to the mothers for whom breastfeeding hasn't gone the way they hoped. We both have had the opportunity to closely walk with dear friends through significant milk supply challenges and we've both shared many a tear with clients for whom we had no answer. Professionally, there is nothing more frustrating to me than unexplained low milk supply, especially when all our efforts, pumping, supplementation, galactogogues, and magic wand waving (!) don't get a family to its goal. Recognizing that a mom's challenges stem from her own health history and exposures, taking it out of the realm of her control, breaks our hearts...and drives us towards finding the solution.

Fortunately, this book provides a wealth of information about a major cause of these struggles for many mothers. Thus far, Insufficient Glandular Tissue (IGT) has been under-researched and poorly understood. This resource shines a light on a number of the factors such as environmental contaminants, the impact of diet, insulin resistance, and maternal BMI that could potentially have an impact on a mother's milk supply...and it recognizes that a "one size fits all" diagnosis and solution isn't possible. I'm a big believer in the adage that "knowledge is power" and I'm grateful that Diana begins to ask the critical questions that will lead us to solid, evidence-based answers for mothers with IGT in the future. While definitive answers are hard to come by, I believe the ideas explored here will lead to significant research in the future that will radically change our understandings about supporting mothers who are struggling with their supplies and expand our options for helping them reach their goals.

I am an IBCLC who is admits that the counseling and support piece of our job comes much easier to me than the nitty-gritty science that makes it all possible. I'm grateful for the breakdown of the science that impacts supply, but the exploration of the lived experiences of mothers with IGT is where my interest is piqued! As an IBCLC who works in a busy lactation practice in Pittsburgh, PA, my greatest take-away from this book is the encouragement to ask a mother what HER goals are when coming face-to-face with the realities of IGT. Helping her to identify what is most important to her--feeding breastmilk or having baby at the breast--feels like an obvious way to support, but one I would not have necessarily thought to explore. I appreciate Diana's clear and understandable guidance for problem solving and creative solutions she provides in this regard.

The other chapter I'm anxious to break-in with constant use is the final one, which highlights resources for use while supporting families in my practice. I appreciate the wide variety of helps including research studies, books, and online resources. We all know that "Googling" IGT won't get us far in regards to quality sources of information, and I'm so grateful for Diana's curation of a guide to reach for when working with families struggling through IGT and other milk supply challenges.

I think this book will be a game-changer in our field. Instead of simply placing a Band-Aid upon the challenge of IGT, we can more thoroughly explore the WHY mothers experience this condition. I believe that it will lead to better solutions and improved outcomes. I'm grateful to know that some mother, somewhere, will read it, or encounter a volunteer or professional who has, and be able to say "I am a breastfeeding mother," where previously there was no hope. Mamas, I believe in you and I'm grateful to have this resource as our guide together.

Amber McCann, IBCLC

Acknowledgements

I've seen so many authors liken the process of writing a book to gestating and giving birth to a child. I'm going add my voice to that chorus by remembering how, before I had my first baby, I thought I knew what being a mother would be all about, but once she arrived, I realized quickly that I had no idea what having a child was like. The same can be said of my journey in writing this book. I've written plenty of things, and I'm a seasoned editor as well, but nothing could have prepared me for the experience of writing, researching, rewriting, reading, revising, and finally submitting this work.

Having been pregnant and given birth three times, I can safely say that I'd rather gestate and give birth than write a book. For starters, pregnancy and birth are on a somewhat predictable time-table. I took more than twice as long to churn out these pages than I thought that I would when I started. Another stark difference between having a child and writing a book is that, ultimately, we arrive at a point of acceptance that we can control only so much of how that child ends up coming out of the womb. We can procreate with someone we think has good genes, take care of ourselves during pregnancy, and give our babies the best shot at a positive transition earthside at birth, but in the end, we know that so much is out of our control. This is not so with a book. Releasing this labor of love has been fraught with more emotional strife than anything else I've ever done. A total career change was less daunting for me than allowing this book to get out there.

Yet this book is not about me at all, and that's what ultimately kept me moving forward to get it written and published. This book is about and for the thousands of mothers around the world for whom lactation didn't go as they wanted or planned. These mothers have shared intimate details about their bodies and their feelings with me, a stranger. I could not have attempted this endeavor without their trust in me; they have gifted me with a perspective I couldn't have obtained otherwise. I hope that this book will empower more mothers than I could ever hope to interact with individually, that they might come to understand, embrace, and overcome the circumstances that brought them to pursue the information within these pages.

As I mention in my introduction, my first inspiration to make the topic of breastfeeding with insufficient glandular tissue my life's work came from my best friend, Heather Shea Greene, to whom this book is dedicated. Heather has been "the wind beneath my wings" for over 20 years, and although her breastfeeding days are behind her, I know she's as happy with the completion of this resource as I am.

I am also forever indebted to the Nelson family, who has given my own family a tremendous gift of friendship and permitted me an intimate look into the realities of breastfeeding with insufficient glandular tissue.

My own family—my husband Bryan and our three children Anna, Simon, and Gabriella—have been immensely patient as this book has consumed many hours over the last 2 years of my life. I've escaped to hotels, missed trips to the zoo, skiing, and hikes…but their pride in me and interest in this project have filled my heart so much. My children think "it's really neat that their mamma wrote a book," and I think they will be very excited to hold a copy in their hands!

Kathy Kendall-Tackett has been a mogul in the breastfeeding education community for longer than I've been part of it. I couldn't have embarked on this journey without her, and I'm incredibly thankful for Kathy's unwavering faith in me and in this book. Her confidence in me represents the bridge between writing and publishing. She's perfectly suited for every hat she wears (and there are many).

Penny Liberatos is mentioned several times in this book because she was my advisor, mentor, and co-investigator while I was earning my Master of Public Health degree and doing research on mothers with lactation insufficiency. Her persistence and insistence on an academic rigor that I hadn't recognized before changed the way I read, write, research, and report. Our research would have been a disaster without her guidance and experience, and this resource would not have been possible without the skills she taught me to develop.

There are many pioneers in the breastfeeding support world who have inspired, encouraged, and supported me during my fledgling years as a La Leche League Leader and International Board Certified Lactation Consultant—too many for me to list (but many are cited in these pages). These women who gave birth to an entire profession come from varied backgrounds, and their unique contributions make this field so rich and full of infinite possibility. We've only just begun to unlock the power of breastfeeding in understanding and improving the entire human race, and I'm proud to fall in behind these pioneers in the long line of lactation support.

Also in the too-many-to-list category are my brilliant colleagues and dear friends in the breastfeeding support community. I would be remiss, however, if I neglected to give a shout-out to my most persistent cheerleaders; Amber McCann, Jeanette McCulloch, Monique Jones, Lara Audelo, and Wendy Bell are always the first to encourage me when I think I can't keep doing this work, often before I've even reached out to them. It's like they know when I need a boost! There are countless more out there who support me with knowledge and love. I consider it a privilege to work with all of you in this noble and vital calling.

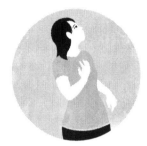

Chapter 1

Why Do I Care About Insufficient Glandular Tissue (IGT)?

Often, we find ourselves pursuing things in our professional lives that represent significant obstacles that we had in our personal lives, but IGT and low milk production were not problems that I encountered at all. Rather, I have had what I consider to be obnoxiously large breasts—large enough that I've considered reduction surgery—almost my entire life, and I struggled with an overproduction of milk with each of my three babies (which opens another entire area of research that I hope to examine someday!).

Heather, my best friend since we were placed on the same Resident Assistant staff during our sophomore year in college, had her first baby in 2006. I had two children at the time. The older weaned (a few months before her fourth birthday) literally days before Heather's daughter was born, and the younger, approaching his second birthday, was still breastfeeding regularly. I had been a La Leche League Leader for a year and was studying and working with mothers and babies under the supervision of a brilliant International Board Certified Lactation Consultant (IBCLC) at a local hospital's mother/baby ward so that I could take the exam to become an IBCLC a few years later.

Heather went into labor earlier than we expected she might, at around 37 weeks, and gave birth to her baby girl by caesarean section for breech presentation. I visited them with dinner in hand and was stricken by how tiny a 5-day-old baby could be. Heather sat for the entire 7 hours that I was there in her comfortable chair with her baby at her breasts. Naturally, I admired my best friend for her tenacity and for not succumbing to the prevailing social pressure to not "spoil the baby." Heather was all too happy to snuggle her little one close and meet her needs at her breasts, breasts that I had never, in our 14 years of friendship, really seen before. Sure, it was sort of a thing between us that I was enormously endowed with DD-cup breasts before I had children and she was constantly in search of the perfect bra that wasn't "bullet-proof," but size didn't matter when it came to breastfeeding, right?

Sitting across the room from my best friend, admiring her baby's perfect latch and Heather's serene comfort—it seemed as if she had been breastfeeding all of her life—my memory burned a little from line drawings and photographs that I had seen months prior of breasts that looked a little different than others I had seen before. Heather's looked like those: tubular, widely spaced, one more than twice the size of the other, with nipples and areolae larger than I would have expected for the size of her breasts.

I didn't know what to say or do in that moment, other than to be relieved that Heather already planned to check in with her pediatrician the next morning for a weight check. Her baby, in the 7 hours that I was there, stayed at Heather's breast but wasn't swallowing very much. She would "suck, suck, suck" for a short while, then fall asleep. I was so early in my own training, but even still, I could recognize an obvious absence of milk transfer. I cried my entire 2-hour drive home, remembering a conversation that I had with my mother during Heather's pregnancy. My mom had asked how Heather was doing, and I told her, "I'm worried about breastfeeding for her, but I'm not really sure why."

What had piqued my interest during Heather's pregnancy was, in fact, the very pregnancy itself. In her second trimester, Heather came to visit me (I was the one with two small children at that time, so traveling was easier for her than for me!), and we marveled over her chart for the cycle in which she got pregnant. It showed that she hadn't really had much of a temperature shift after her cervical fluid had dried up. Even later in her luteal phase, there was no characteristic triphasic temperature pattern that would indicate the ovulatory phase, ovulation and the resultant warming progesterone secretion from the corpus luteum, and the implantation of the embryo, which, for many women, causes another perceptible rise in basal body temperature. Heather had often spotted before her period, and she did so in her early pregnancy as well. I could tell from her chart that her progesterone levels were not robust, although they were obviously high enough to sustain her pregnancy that cycle.

"So, when does the booby fairy arrive?" Heather asked me. She was well into her second trimester and was a glowing, gorgeous pregnant woman. But, after waiting her entire adult life for the gift of breasts that was purported to accompany pregnancy, she was disappointed when it seemed the booby fairy had somehow missed her house.

"You didn't feel anything at all? No heat, tingling, nothing?" I asked her, remembering the sensation of my swollen, ponderous breasts on fire, as if they might explode right there on my chest. "Um, I don't think so. When was it supposed to happen?" Heather was curious. I didn't remember for sure, but I did know that by the time I was into my second trimester, I was already busting out of new bras and maternity clothes.

When I got home after spending the day with Heather and her newborn, I emailed a few La Leche League Leader/IBCLC friends who could point me in the direction of some resources. At the time, I was helping review an initial draft of Diana West and Lisa Marasco's (2008), *The Breastfeeding Mother's Guide to Making More Milk,* and I had been researching low milk production for a little over a year on behalf of my friend Renee. But without developed research skills or even keywords, my searches were rather futile. I read every major lactation resource that I could get my hands on, but there was only the occasional mention of breasts that had specific physical characteristics and didn't manage to produce adequate milk. Other than in *The Breastfeeding Mother's Guide to Making More Milk* (which hadn't even yet been published—I still marvel at the blessing it was for me to have been even minimally involved, at that very time, in a resource that I knew would be so valuable!), there was little guidance on how to actually help these mothers. Just a sort of unwritten shrug and head nod that acknowledged, reluctantly, that not every mother could breastfeed.

I felt almost as if this information was held in secret. Even just a decade ago, when I began breastfeeding my own child, breastfeeding was less common than it is now, and the assertion that breastfeeding is a public health issue, not a lifestyle choice, was not yet widely accepted. The field of lactation is still relatively new. La Leche League emerged only in the late 1950s, and the International Board of Lactation Consultant Examiners (IBLCE),

Finding Sufficiency

the certifying body for IBCLCs, was founded in 1985. Even so, its scholars in the lactation field have done remarkable things to support breastfeeding mothers without a foundational body of academically vetted evidence on which to base some practices. These are women (with a handful of talented male IBCLCs as well) with diverse, often non-health care backgrounds that recognize the need for clinical support for breastfeeding. Earning the respect of the medical community at large has been an uphill battle.

The body of evidence used to create and support protocols and practice is growing rapidly, and the accessibility of information today is remarkable thanks to the Internet and social media. Still, many on the frontlines of support for new mothers are not exposed to important new findings. Without concrete diagnostic criteria for IGT, health care providers are left to work in a gray area where nothing is definite. We can look at a pregnant woman's breasts and see asymmetry, a tubular shape, and a small amount of breast tissue stuffed into bulging nipples. Yet we can't say, "you have a 61% chance of not being able to fully breastfeed your baby," on the basis of one study (Huggins, Petok, & Mireles, 2000) or without knowledge of other risk and protective factors for that particular mother's milk production capabilities.

Heather sought guidance from her breastfeeding-friendly pediatrician, who told her to "keep at it" and didn't really acknowledge that not producing enough milk was even a possibility. Her prenatal health care practice included midwives and an obstetrician (OB) that supported normal birth but had nothing to offer her in terms of her breasts. To our horror, the local IBCLC that she sought out and visited had never heard the term mammary hypoplasia. We were left with…me. Feeling grossly underequipped, I was thankful when someone else gave Heather an at-breast supplementing device and showed her how to use it. The thought of pumping was unappealing to her, so Heather supplemented with formula and felt a mix of relief and devastation when her baby thrived on it and finally began to grow. In the end, with the help of some herbs, she made just over half of the milk her baby needed, but she deeply and truly enjoyed their breastfeeding relationship. Their breastfeeding experience continued, and she did not need supplementation after the first year, "like a normal mother," until her child was past her second birthday.

Naturally, I learned a great deal about breastfeeding with low milk production from a clinical perspective through Heather's experience. But the bigger eye-opener for me was the emotional roller coaster that Heather had to ride through her baby's first year, wondering if she had done something wrong, not knowing anyone else who had this problem, feeling like she wouldn't be welcome at breastfeeding support groups because she also gave her baby formula, worrying when there was a national recall on the formula brand she was using, and experiencing guilt and frustration when her baby needed nebulizer treatments to help her breathe. Did this happen because she didn't have enough breastmilk to feed her exclusively?

She experienced isolation when well-meaning family, friends, and even health care providers told her that "breastfeeding wasn't that big a deal, anyway"; despair (or was it validation?) when her baby totally refused a bottle once they finally got the hang of supplementing at the breast; and immense joy when she looked down at her sweet, blue-eyed toddler smiling up at her while she had her "ni-nighs" before sleeping. When we know our experience isn't the way that we imagine everyone else's to be, every bump in the road, whether other mothers are experiencing it or not, feels like it's attributable to our particular problem. The emotional cost of breastfeeding with IGT is often as complicated (or even more so) as the logistical obstacles.

It's this emotional cost that I seek to mitigate by publishing this book. I have repeatedly seen the triumphs of mothers who've come to understand and accept how their breastfeeding expectations were not fulfilled. They triumphed in the end because they claimed the aspects of lactation and mothering that were most important to them from the start and maximized them within the physical confines with they dealt. Rather than having a bitter vendetta against breastfeeding and all who support it, mothers who become victorious over IGT are informed and empowered.

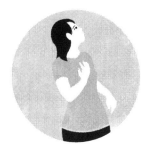

Chapter 2

An Introduction to IGT

IGT is relatively rare. There are other, more likely causes for low milk output in mothers who intend to exclusively breastfeed their babies and have the social and clinical support to do so. Yet I believe that each mother who discovers that she has it, often after being unable to exclusively meet her newborn baby's nutritional needs with her milk alone, is one too many. There are few resources available to help mothers and practitioners understand what IGT is, who might have it, and what kind of help can be given to those with it.

I aim to fill a gap for mothers and those who support them, including obstetricians who see mothers during the prenatal and immediate postnatal periods, midwives, pediatricians, and lactation consultants. Practitioners can glean important knowledge and practical tools for seeing their breastfeeding patients with IGT through the confusion and heartbreak of lactation insufficiency.

Through the generosity of over 1,300 mothers around the world, I will share clinical knowledge and data about IGT and the mothers who may have it and, hopefully, help each reader chart her own course toward triumph over this unexpected condition. This resource is not a how-to. I won't tell you how to increase your milk supply, though more milk might result from a better understanding of your situation. I'm not going to tell you how to feed your baby, but you might find ideas that you didn't think of and resources to help you carry out the decisions you make.

Mothers with IGT are a subset of a larger population: mothers with low milk production. This book presumes that you have already assessed, thoroughly and with the help of appropriate professionals, other possible causes for low milk production. Diana West, IBCLC, and Lisa Marasco, M.A., IBCLC, authored a comprehensive resource in 2008 for those who are still examining maternal and infant factors that may contribute to difficulty producing milk. I consider their book, *The Breastfeeding Mother's Guide to Making More Milk,* to be a prerequisite to this resource. Most milk-making issues are more readily resolved than IGT. If yours is among those addressed in *The Breastfeeding Mother's Guide to Making More Milk,* you can find solutions there. This book is for those who feel certain, after ruling out all other maternal or infant causes for low milk supply, that their milk production challenge is due to insufficient glandular development of one or both breasts. Chapter 3 provides some solid information to help you determine whether your breastfeeding difficulties can be attributed to IGT.

The lactation support community is often frustrated by the profound dearth of studies that help them understand and manage breastfeeding difficulties. This lack of research may lead many mothers to wean their babies prematurely and falling short of the U.S. *Healthy People 2020* goals for exclusive breastfeeding: 46.2% of babies exclusively breastfeeding (no other food or drink but mother's milk) at 3 months and 25.5% of babies exclusively breastfeeding at 6 months (U.S. Department of Health and Human Services [HHS], 2012).

Significant strides are being made in areas such as tongue tie and lip tie (lingual and labial frenula) assessment and treatment, better hospital management of birth and breastfeeding, and access to professional lactation support. IBCLCs are becoming more available in the United States, as the Patient Protection and Affordable Care Act (health care reform, or "Obamacare") offers provisions for mothers to receive this important aspect of postpartum care. However, there is little information, other than that which we acquire through our clinical practice or can piece together from other factors in a mother's appearance and history, that pertains directly to breastfeeding with IGT. There seems, instead, to be an attitude of "well, there's always formula," which may be true, but really sells short the commitment and capability of mothers to give their babies a start to life that is as biologically normal as possible, even if that means less than 100% breastfeeding.

In this book, I cite research, but much of the material I present comes directly from clinical exposure to mothers who have shared their experiences with me. I hope that this "practice-based evidence," combined with the support from the literature we do have, will allow mothers and their supporters to tap into the collective wisdom of those who have worked with their physiological challenges and gone on to have fulfilling breastfeeding relationships.

Perhaps the most important of these hundreds of mothers are two of my dearest friends. Each is truly the kind of friend we hope we're fortunate enough to meet and have in our lives. As I described in the Introduction, Heather had her first baby in 2006 and struggled to breastfeed with IGT. The experience of being a devoted breastfeeding advocate, breastfeeding mother, IBCLC-to-be, and Heather's best friend all at the same time blew my mind and, although I didn't know it at the time, changed the course of my life. While being privy to her searing emotions of anger, frustration, guilt, confusion, and betrayal, I was exposed—about as close to firsthand as I could possibly be without actually being unable to breastfeed—to a rather dark side of breastfeeding support, a side that no one in the medical community seemed to acknowledge.

My earlier experience with lactation failure was with my friend Renee, who when we met was struggling with immense shame and self-loathing every time she bottle-fed her infant with a breastmilk substitute. Her first baby was a few months younger than mine, and we connected during the second half of our babies' first year. We were both having a hard time: she with her feeding struggles and me with my own attachment parenting stigma: separation from my baby when I had to go to work. Renee and I shared worries that every challenge we had with our babies was because we couldn't do mothering exactly the way it was "supposed to be done."

After a less-than-optimal birth experience and start to breast-feeding, Renee sought the very best breastfeeding support that was available in the metro New York area at the time. She had grown weary of other mothers at playgroups and on Internet forums who suggested that maybe she hadn't *really* tried *everything* and that being unable to breastfeed was somehow her fault. Renee shared her full history with me slowly, over a few years. By the time she was planning for the arrival of her second baby in 2007, I had been exposed to a lot more information and was fervently researching on her (and Heather's) behalf. Although Renee had a much more positive breastfeeding experience the second time around, the measures that she and her husband took, the money they spent, and the effort they put forth to feed their baby, about half with Renee's milk and half with donor milk from other mothers (when they could get it; this was before the emergence of mother-to-mother milk sharing as a common practice), gave me a very close reminder of the reality that, for mothers with IGT, breastfeeding and lactation are anything but easy. In addition, the experience of breastfeeding (for all mothers) is about so much more than the protective and health-promoting aspects of feeding human milk to a human baby.

As the public health message about the importance of breast-feeding grows and becomes more widely accepted around the globe, we are seeing increased "intention" to breastfeed, and we are learning more about providing "social support" for that intention. Yet our capacity to support women for whom lactation fails is not keeping pace with the growing numbers of mothers who are choosing to breastfeed their babies and are seeking help and support to do so.

As I have already stated, there is very little evidence with regard to IGT upon which to draw. I am indebted to the mothers who have so generously and candidly shared their experiences and medical histories with me. Of particular note are the mothers who belonged to an email list called *Not Everyone Can Breastfeed*, which is run by an IGT mom, Heather Wong, and the women who continue to come together on the Facebook IGT and Low Milk Supply Support Group. The administrators of that group, Nyssa Retter, Jessica Butanda, Melissa Letham, Lauren Wu, and Brandy Mitchell (and now Kelly Duxfield and Rachael Lawrence Fisher) devoted—and continue to devote—countless hours to collating information and moderating conversations that are, understandably, often emotionally charged. The mothers in that Facebook group and those who participated in my thesis research (with my co-investigator, Dr. Penny Liberatos) are invested in enabling other mothers to have an easier time of breastfeeding than they had, and without their collective voices, I would have only my own undeveloped speculation to share.

The mothers' voices you will read in this book are quotes from real women who participated in my thesis research. Those who've experienced breastfeeding problems will feel right at home with those excerpts, but other readers may feel shocked or surprised by the anger and frustration that is expressed in them. It is time for the lactation support community to embrace that there may be *circumstances of our modern times*—environmental influences, diet over time, and disease states—that make human lactation a less stable, less reliable process of our biology than it had to be in order for our species to be sustained in previous millennia.

I am of the mind that breastfeeding and lactation, which ideally go together, are different (albeit closely related) functions of motherhood. A mother may learn that her ability to lactate is compromised, but this doesn't have to mean that the transformative experience of mothering through breastfeeding is lost for her. In this book, I aim to provide the encouragement and practical support that mothers with IGT need as they adjust and pursue their personal breastfeeding goals.

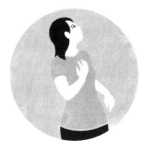

Chapter 3

Do I Have IGT?

For most mothers, even those with breastfeeding difficulties, the answer to this question is no. In fact, you may conclude, after reading this book and learning that not all cases of lactation failure are caused by insufficient glandular development, that you don't actually have IGT (Chapters 5 and 6 will still be valuable to you, so keep reading!). For the majority of mothers with truly insufficient milk output to exclusively breastfeed, something else more likely went wrong. These problems could include:

- Problems with breastfeeding management, such as parents or caregivers trying to schedule feeds, using a pacifier to space feeds out, or limiting the amount of time that baby spends at the breast

- Something about the baby that makes it difficult for him to suck properly, stimulate your breasts, and transfer milk, such as tongue tie or an orofacial cleft

- Hormonal issues that make a mother's full complement of glandular tissue less able to function properly for lactation

> *I am still stunned at how painful it is to read how "rare" this condition is. It does not feel rare to me when I am experiencing it. I feel dismissed and that women who are successfully breastfeeding think I am making excuses.*

Lactation failure is a phrase I don't like to use, but I'm at a loss for how else to describe the inability of a mother to put out enough milk, either through direct breastfeeding or expression, so that her baby may be fed only his mother's milk for the first 6 months of his life. I struggle with the phrase *lactation failure* because I believe that any milk output is wonderful, and if there is any milk at all, isn't that lactation, albeit "incomplete lactation"?

Alison Stuebe, MD, MSc, a maternal–fetal medicine specialist and breastfeeding researcher, has coined the colloquial term *lacta-tastrophe* to describe these "lactation catastrophes." Unfortunately, because of the lack of definitive literature on this topic, we are stuck, for now, with *lactation failure*. When I refer to this, I really do mean "incomplete lactation."

> *I use an at-breast supplementer. I love my baby, she is my world. We have a breastfeeding relationship. I may not be able to exclu-sively breastfeed but what I can give her means the world to me.*

Lactation failure can be classified into three categories: preglan-dular, glandular, and postglandular (Morton, 1994). Because most difficulties in lactation can be traced to postglandular issues, let's cover those first. Postglandular causes of insufficient milk output are those things that happen after the baby is born that get breast-feeding off to a bad start, such as a baby who cannot properly transfer milk at the breast or where there is poor breastfeeding management, such as scheduled feeds or the extended separation of mother and baby.

The vast majority of milk production problems are of a postglan-dular nature. Even though a lot is known about these problems, not all practitioners are able to identify or assist in dealing with them. In fact, those practitioners we trust to help us can be the ones who steer us in the wrong direction with well-intentioned but misguided advice. Many mothers lament, months after their breastfeeding experiences ended prematurely, they wish someone had told them that something was actually wrong and interfering with normal lactation.

> For me, it was absolutely devastating to be incapable of making enough milk for my children. While I was pregnant with my first I dreamed about being a mom—and always motherhood was represented by breastfeeding. To be unable to "properly" do so was very difficult. Additionally there was NO information available (volunteered) to me from the six IBCLCs, three OBs, three midwives, and two pediatricians I went to over the course of my children, which suggested that I might have IGT. It was only after reading about it and then bringing it to a practitioner's attention was it confirmed that I did have IGT.

Ankyloglossia, or tongue tie, is one condition that seems to be on the rise in babies, particularly the often-missed posterior tongue ties. These are not immediately obvious to the untrained eye but can restrict the baby's ability to move his tongue and feed properly.

A tongue tied baby may have difficulty transferring milk from the breast, and this can result in inadequate stimulation of the mother's breasts. This sets up a domino effect, which, for a mother with a normal complement of glandular tissue, might present a bump in the road but one that can be overcome with assistance and the appropriate protocols for stimulating additional milk production.

Even if a doctor, nurse, or lactation consultant looked at your baby's oral anatomy and told you that "everything was fine," it is still possible that a tongue tie was at least partly a cause of your milk production issues.

Just like many otherwise competent professionals do not recognize IGT, it is possible that competent health care providers may not recognize tongue tie or recommend treatment for it. Books and websites that offer more information about tongue tie are listed in the Resource Chapter of this book.

Preglandular Causes

Preglandular causes for low or no milk production are directly related to hormonal issues, such as a retained placenta, a known (or unknown) endocrine disorder, or postpartum thyroiditis.

Often, mothers who think their milk production issues are due to IGT also (or only) have a preglandular cause for their lactation failure. These preglandular causes for poor lactation outcomes can be particularly problematic in women who also have IGT. An undiagnosed tongue tie, for example, can create a problem that might be difficult or impossible to recover from: the mother might have never had the potential to make a full milk supply, but her milk-making potential will be stunted that much further by the undiagnosed tongue tie. This is in part because, in the early postpartum days/weeks, lactation is driven by a complex hormonal process.

This process is wonderfully designed. At the time when a newborn baby wants only to suckle at his mother's breast, the mother's anatomy requires that frequent suckling to stimulate multiple, frequent prolactin spikes. These prolactin spikes in the immediate postpartum period promote the development of prolactin receptors in the breasts. The more receptors there are, the better the mother's body will be able to use the smaller amounts of prolactin that are available when milk production becomes less hormonally driven (endocrine) and more supply-and-demand driven (autocrine).

If frequent, adequate stimulation to the breasts does not take place in those early postpartum weeks, the foundation for future milk production may be compromised.

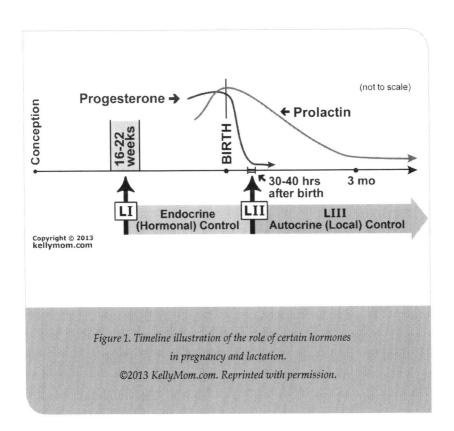

Figure 1. Timeline illustration of the role of certain hormones
in pregnancy and lactation.
©2013 KellyMom.com. Reprinted with permission.

Hormone dysfunction can be multilayered, in that the hormonal setting during adolescence, when the breasts should be developing, might set the stage for lactation failure many years later. Certain hormonal problems in puberty may impair glandular development as well (Marasco, Marmet, & Shell, 2000), and/or the current hormonal setting is inhibiting what glandular tissue did develop (whether it was a full complement or not), thereby preventing it from reaching its full potential for making milk.

It can be confusing to think of hormones in terms of both how they affect glandular *development* (whether your breasts grow and change during puberty and pregnancy) and how they affect glandular *behavior*. So here, we'll focus on glandular development. West and Marasco (2008) discussed the effects of thyroid, androgens, and polycystic ovarian syndrome (PCOS) on lactation—glandular behavior—in their book, *The Breastfeeding Mother's Guide to Making More Milk*. If you have or suspect endocrine dysfunction, understanding that and working with a qualified health care provider to normalize what's going on in your individual body is very important.

Glandular Causes for Low Milk Output

IGT—a lack of milk-making tissue in the breasts—is a glandular cause of an inability to produce enough milk to breastfeed exclusively. Let me reiterate that glandular causes of lactation insufficiency are often complicated by preglandular and postglandular causes. However, in many cases, even a glandular obstacle that exists by itself, without other causes, is only surmountable to a point. Other breastfeeding problems can often be overcome completely with appropriate, qualified support. Some mothers with slight IGT, perhaps with ample, dense tissue in three quadrants of the breast, might be able to attain a full milk supply, but many will not, no matter what is done.

Glandular causes for low or no milk production can include previous breast or chest surgery. While these won't always compromise lactation and they are rarely a surprise (most mothers know they've had surgery in that area and that it might affect breastfeeding), the struggles that can accompany these causes are real. The authoritative resource for breastfeeding after surgery is Diana West's (2001), *Defining Your Own Success: Breastfeeding After Breast Reduction Surgery.* Her resource also includes strategies for those experiencing other types of lactation failure, whether they are preglandular or glandular in nature.

Hypoplasia or IGT?

There may be some confusion between the terms *hypoplasia* and *IGT* because they are often used interchangeably. *Hypoplasia* is a term used to describe an organ—any part of the body—that hasn't fully developed. When we are speaking about breasts, we use the terms *mammary hypoplasia* to refer to the underdeveloped mammary glands or *breast hypoplasia* to talk about the underdevelopment of the breasts. Underdevelopment of one or both breasts, characterized by particular physical markers (which will be described further in this chapter) may suggest (but not exclusively predict!) milk-making difficulty and a functional inability to produce enough milk to exclusively breastfeed a baby. In other words, the *appearance* of hypoplastic breasts may have no bearing whatsoever on their function.

From a diagnostic perspective, our ability to assess for and characterize hypoplasia does not clearly lead us to a subsequent prediction of lactation insufficiency. It only gives us a name for what we can see about the breasts. Similarly, the physical characteristics of hypoplasia may be masked, especially in women with a prepregnant body mass index (BMI) greater than 30, such that we think we're looking at voluptuous, bountiful breasts that should be overflowing with milk, but they don't because all the big bra size reflects is adipose or fatty tissue.

In this book, I use the term IGT to describe breasts that have compromised function because of incomplete glandular development because we are dealing with *known insufficiency.* We are talking about breasts that do not readily make enough milk for exclusive breastfeeding.

> *I'm not in the norm for IGT, in that I have large breasts ... but breast size alone is not enough to indicate presence of IGT. I wish that the medical profession would take this more seriously, and educate themselves so that they in turn could help women who might not know that IGT even exists.*

Another important factor to note is that, for some women, one breast takes on a clearly hypoplastic appearance and/or function, but the other breast looks normal (keeping in mind that there is a wide range of what a "normal" breast might look like), functions perfectly well—perhaps even makes a full milk supply. Many mothers refer to their "good" breasts with words like *champ, superboob, producer, big milky,* and *tweedle-dee* (yes, really!) and offer less flattering, maybe not so politically correct words like *dud, gimpy, lazy-daisy,* and *tweedle-dumb* to describe the breasts that don't work so well. (As an aside, I like to encourage mothers to use kind words when thinking or speaking about their breasts or any part of their bodies. Isn't there enough judgment and negativity in the world already? We don't need to heap it on ourselves, even when we feel that our bodies betray us.)

Because asymmetry is one marker of insufficient glandular development, a corresponding disparity in milk output is very common among mothers with IGT. It bears noting, though, that even mothers without milk-making issues might have one breast that produces significantly more milk than the other, so this factor alone can't tell us we're dealing with IGT.

> Not all women with IGT have both breasts affected. Some of us have one breast that hardly produces any milk, but the other breast doubles in size, making us completely lopsided. Although this is wonderful for the baby and breastfeeding, I felt very unsure of myself. What did my husband think? How does the world perceive me? Am I a freak? None of these are good thoughts and although breastfeeding is wonderful, it has been a rollercoaster of happy days and very sad and depressing days. The joys of sitting with one breast having an "over abundant supply" and the other one having very low supply.

References to underdeveloped breasts, with or without noted lactation failure, can be found in ancient texts. Does this mean hypoplasia is not a new condition? The plastic surgery literature has included references to tubular breasts for nearly 40 years, but these references address appearance, not breast function or lactation capability.

The first known reference to lactation failure related to breast appearance was in 1985, when Neifert, Seacat, and Jobe documented the lactation experiences of three women with normal prolactin levels and adequate breast stimulation. In the nearly 30 years since their publication, we still have these important words at the forefront of our discourse of lactation failure due to insufficient glandular development:

> It is suggested that, although the vast majority of women can nurse successfully, the breast, like every other organ, experiences functional failure. Suggestive history and physical findings may be clues to the detection of insufficient glandular development among a small number of women who will be unable to fully breastfeed, despite the most heroic efforts. Confirmation and appropriate explanation are warranted to dispel guilt feelings and to prevent failure to thrive in subsequent infants. Breast-feeding [sic] can continue with a high degree of maternal satisfaction and infant well-being by supplementing with formula via the Lact-Aid device or by bottle (p. 828).

Neifert et al. (1985) also mentioned a large prospective study that was being planned to determine the actual incidence of lactation failure associated with insufficient glandular development, but major centers for lactation study at that time were unable to recruit enough mothers who met the criteria for the study. This led to the now-infamous (but undocumentable) assumption that up to 5% of mothers may experience primary lactation failure. Some argue that this number is too small and that the actual number of women with IGT is much higher. Others believe that the actual cause of low milk production in the majority of these cases that appear to be hypoplasia is endocrine (hormone-related) and can be remedied sufficiently that a mother, with the proper guidance, could produce enough milk.

Because there are so many criteria—many of them subjective—surrounding the inability to breastfeed, it is possible that we may never be able to more definitively state what the percentage of insurmountable lactation failure truly is. Is there a standard by which we can determine whether a mother "did everything" or "tried hard enough" in order to earn such a diagnosis? I don't believe there is—or should be. One mother may have expended hours of effort each day coaxing her breasts to eke out enough that her baby thrived on her milk alone. Did she have IGT? Her lactation experience was not physiologically normal or stable. What about the mother who chose to mixed-feed her baby so that she could spend her time preserving the calm, close moments of nurturing her baby at her breasts? Did she "try hard enough"? Did she have IGT? We know that her lactation experience wasn't physiologically normal or stable either. We may never really know the true prevalence of IGT in the population.

> *Finding out after four years that my inability to nurse my children was not my fault was both devastating and liberating—I could*

throw off the guilt that burdened me through my first three nursing experiences and finally become proactive in finding a real solution that would help me and my next baby to have a healthy, loving, guilt-free nursing relationship.

A major breakthrough in the understanding of the possible relationship between breast appearance and function was made upon the publication of the only study to date that has examined it. In 2000, Huggins, Petok, & Mireles published "Markers of Lactation Insufficiency: A Study of 34 Mothers," in *Current Issues in Clinical Lactation.* Their findings suggested that the following characteristics may be correlated with an inability to produce enough breastmilk to exclusively meet the nutritional needs of a breastfeeding baby:

- Tubular or constricted breast shape, with breasts occupying a shorter space on the chest (covering the third through fifth ribs rather than the second through sixth)

- Widely spaced breasts (with more than 1.5 inches between breasts)

- Stretch marks

- Obvious asymmetry between the two breasts

- Little or no breast changes during pregnancy

- No engorgement or feeling of "milk coming in" postpartum

While the Huggins et al. study did establish a relationship between these markers and difficulty producing milk, the markers were not shown to be 100% predictive of future milk-making trouble; 39% of mothers (12 of the 34) went on to produce enough milk for their babies after 1 month. Larger studies are definitely called for, but the findings of this one may be enough to justify prenatal breast assessment by health care providers and increased awareness of the relationship between these physical characteristics and the potential for milk production troubles.

> *It was devastating. And it feels singular and lonely. There are far too few resources, studies etc. on this subject. Why didn't anyone in my 31 years look at my breasts and say "hey, you have similar characteristics of this condition. Let's talk about it."*

What Is Insufficient?

The terms that plastic surgeons use to describe breasts that have not fully developed include:

- Tuberous breast deformity (or simply tuberous or tubular breasts)

- Snoopy breasts (yes, really!)

- Constricted breasts

- Hypoplastic breasts

The word *insufficient* is a controversial one: insufficient for…what? The bulk of the literature about underdeveloped breasts addresses appearance, not function. Many readers of this book likely have breasts that, if the standard is filling a bra cup or shaping a sweater against your body, are quite "sufficient," but do not make enough milk to exclusively feed a baby. Matters are complicated further when the term IGT is used because the actual amount of glandular tissue that is needed to produce a full milk supply varies widely between mothers.

These breasts, if seen separately, might not appear hypoplastic, but when they are viewed together, we see asymmetry, a tubular shape, and wide spacing. They are not small breasts.

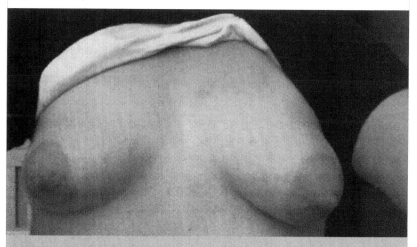

Figure 2. Used with permission of anonymous contributor. Photo may not be reproduced.

This is the appearance of what many would call a classic presentation of hypoplasia: asymmetry, very wide spacing, stretch marks where there was no growth, and no breast changes during pregnancy. However, it is worth nothing that this mother, with the assistance of herbal products that acted on her blood sugar and insulin sensitivity, was able to meet her baby's nutritional needs almost exclusively. Appearance can't tell us everything we need to know.

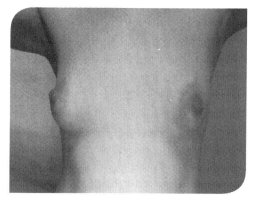

Figure 3. Used with permission of anonymous contributor. Photo may not be reproduced.

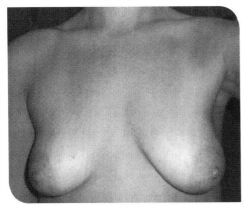

Here is another example of breasts that, if seen only one at a time, might appear perfectly normal but, seen together, show subtle asymmetry, stretch marks, moderately wide spacing, and nipples that turn outward, which are suggestive of a lack of dense glandular tissue in the lower middle sections of each breast.

Figure 4. Used with permission of anonymous contributor. Photo may not be reproduced.

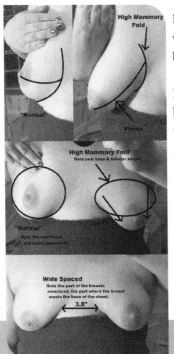

Note the characteristic tubular shape, wide spacing, and asymmetry of these breasts.

For additional real-life photos of IGT breasts that struggled to produce milk, visit IGT mom Nyssa Retter's blog, *Diary of a Lactation Failure.*

Her post *"The Many Faces (Well, Not Faces) of IGT"* (*http://diaryofalactationfail-ure.blogspot.com/2011/12/many-faces-well-not-faces-of-igt.html*) is a virtual gallery of IGT breasts.

You might find your "boob twin" there!

Figure 5. © 2013 Brandy Mitchell. Reprinted with permission.

This is where we get the whole "size doesn't matter" argument, which is valid in most cases. Breasts with a certain ratio of glandular to fat tissue in one woman may make lots of milk, whereas the same or even greater ratio of glandular to fat tissue may exist in another mother whose breasts make very little milk. The difference may be in the hormonal situation the mother is in, whether her endocrine system supports lactation or works against it; or even whether her hormones were doing what they were supposed to during the time her breasts should have been developing.

Many mothers wonder whether an ultrasound image or some other means of looking inside of their breasts might offer a definitive diagnosis of IGT. Neifert et al. (1985) suggested that breast diaphranography might be a valuable tool, but no method of examining the composition of breasts has been predictive of future milk output. Breast diaphranography is the use of a noninvasive imaging procedure for the detection and evaluation of breast disease. It uses the visualization and comparison of the density of breast tissue through a television camera that is sensitive to infrared light. There is no magic ratio of glandular tissue to fat tissue, no known specific mass of glandular tissue that is necessary to meet the needs of a baby.

One study attempted to correlate breast composition with milk output with ultrasound imaging (Ramsay, Kent, Hartmann, & Hartmann, 2005), but the amount or ratio of glandular tissue and fat tissue in the breasts were not predictive of lactation outcomes. While imaging may provide information about how much of the breast is actually fat versus glandular, it tells us nothing about what that glandular tissue is capable of doing under the right conditions. Simply put, breast composition alone doesn't predict the ability (or inability) to produce milk. We can observe physical markers in the presence of insufficient milk output, but even then, conclusive diagnostic means for IGT development are slippery and evasive.

I want to know if I can definitively get it diagnosed.

We can also ask: who can provide this diagnosis? Hypoplastic-appearing breasts are often first recognized by an IBCLC, but it is not within the scope of practice for a lactation consultant (unless she is also a physician or nurse practitioner) to provide a diagnosis or prescribe treatment.

An IBCLC can only document what she sees and either share those observations with the client's health care provider or encourage the mother to do so herself. For example, although an IBCLC shouldn't declare, "you have hypoplasia," she might describe the mother's breasts or note the following on a report:

> Breasts are spaced 2.5 inches apart, and asymmetry is obvious, with left breast appearing two cup sizes larger than right breast. Left breast is tubular in shape. Both nipple/areolar complexes appear bulbous, perhaps suggestive of minimal breast tissue present and herniated into nipple. Per Huggins, Petok, and Mireles (2000), these physical characteristics may be indicative of mammary hypoplasia or insufficient glandular development for lactation and a risk factor for low milk output.

A definitive diagnosis for why certain breasts can't produce milk is difficult to pin down. Yet this is what so many mothers who aren't able to exclusively breastfeed their babies so desperately want: a diagnosis. Although there are diagnostic codes for lactation dysfunction or lactation failure, these obviously are general and provide little basis for how to proceed with treatment or prevention. Culturally, mothers who don't produce enough milk for their babies encounter criticism from family, friends, other mothers, and medical providers. They may also perceive that they are being criticized in the media and via health promotion messages. A diagnosis might serve as a trump card in the face of all of that criticism, all of those doubts about whether the mother "tried hard enough" or "really tried everything." But the ability to make this diagnosis remains elusive.

Encouraging mothers to focus more on what is going well or right rather than on what has failed or gone wrong is an important aspect of counseling and care when IGT is a possible culprit. But it doesn't take away mothers' desires to name what went wrong with the breastfeeding relationships that they thought they were going to have.

> I've had very little support from the medical field. Most doctors and child health nurses know very little about it. More education is needed. Lots of times I often got dismissed from lactation consultants. They didn't believe that I didn't have enough milk and that I wasn't trying enough. It was really disheartening when I was feeding hourly around the clock, pumping in-between feeds, taking supplements and teas, and eating well. I would often just

get told to keep feeding and I was doing well. I just ended up frustrated and confused. Having recognition and acceptance has been a huge relief for me and has given me confidence to continue to keep trying to breastfeed along with supplementing.

The attribution of milk production issues to glandular insufficiency is a "conclusion of exclusion," one we can come to when we've got certain physical and functional markers that may be (and often are) complicated by other factors. What is important to consider is that, while yes, problems in the early days and weeks can affect milk production in the long term, mothers with no hormonal issues and a "full complement" (whatever that means) of glandular tissue will usually rebound after 72 hours of good, purposeful breast stimulation if the problem (such as a tongue tie in the baby or the overuse of a pacifier) is detected and addressed early enough in the postpartum period. Milk production that continues to lag even after proper management, in the presence of these physical and functional markers, may be due to IGT. Keeping in mind that preglandular and postglandular factors often account for some of the milk deficit, when we normalize hormones and properly stimulate the breasts of a mother who truly has IGT, we're still only going to get what we're going to get.

It is heartbreaking to have the "right of breastfeeding" taken away from you by your own body. But it's comforting to know why it happened and to know that you aren't the only one. It's also weirdly gratifying to be able to put people in their place when they blame you for your lack of milk. You can tell them that THEY are wrong, you have an actual disorder beyond "not trying hard enough."

How Do I Know if IGT Is Really My Problem?

In the absence of a consensus on how we might classify lactation insufficiency as caused by IGT, I use the following criteria to identify IGT cases:

- Intent to exclusively breastfeed from birth through the middle of the baby's first year (about 6 months)

- Appropriate social and clinical support for the intent to breastfeed, resulting in proper breastfeeding management and early detection/resolution of any infant difficulties in breast stimulation or milk transfer

- Lack of breast changes in pregnancy (breasts did not become at all sensitive, warm/hot, swollen, or larger in size during early pregnancy)

- Lack of or "spotty" breast changes postpartum (some mothers feel "engorgement" where they do have glandular tissue, typically in all quadrants except the lower middle quadrant)

- A medically indicated need to feed a supplement other than mother's milk to the baby within the first 14 days after birth[1]

- Widely spaced breasts or nipples that seem to "look away" from each other or "look down," which indicate soft, fatty tissue in the lower center quadrant of the breasts

- Asymmetrical breasts

---

1   This can be subjective. Normal newborn infant behavior is often poorly understood, and it is common for health care providers and parents to misinterpret normal newborn needs for physical closeness and suckling as hunger. Every effort should be made by qualified practitioners and parents to distinguish between normal newborn behavior and insufficient nutrition in the first 2 weeks of life.

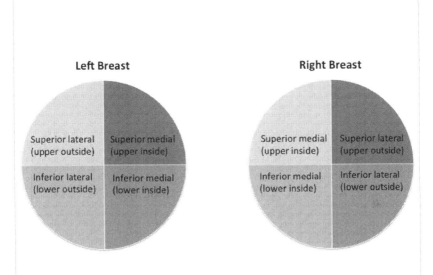

Left Breast   **Right Breast**

| Superior lateral (upper outside) | Superior medial (upper inside) |
| Inferior lateral (lower outside) | Inferior medial (lower inside) |

| Superior medial (upper inside) | Superior lateral (upper outside) |
| Inferior medial (lower inside) | Inferior lateral (lower outside) |

Figure 6. Diagram of the breast quadrants. In clinical observations, most often, mothers can feel an absence of glandular tissue in the inferior medial (lower inside) quadrants.

This may cause that area of the breast to be flaccid compared with the quadrants that hold dense glandular tissue. This results in breasts that "sag" or nipples that, if they were eyes, might "look away" from each other or "look down." This may also contribute to the wide spacing that accompanies breasts with a hypoplastic appearance.

Clinicians should always assess both breasts at the same time from a distance about halfway across the room (5–10 feet at least) when they evaluate a patient for IGT markers.

Remember that appearance alone cannot predict future lactational function of the breasts.

In 2013, Penny Liberatos (New York Medical College) and I conducted a study of mothers with breastfeeding difficulties related to milk supply.

As a result of that research, we determined that other red flags that might be present in mothers with IGT include:

- A prepregnant body mass index (BMI) of greater than 30

- BMI greater than 26 or 30 during puberty

- Hormonal disorders, such as insulin resistance, diabetes, or hyperandrogenism

- Use of hormonal birth control during puberty (for reasons other than to prevent pregnancy)

- Unexplained fertility issues

- History of an eating disorder or extreme athleticism that delayed or stopped menstruation

However, even in Huggins et al.'s sample, there were women with the physical presentation of hypoplasia/IGT who made enough milk to exclusively breastfeed, and there are women with very full-appearing breasts who make barely any milk after their babies are born. How can you determine if IGT is really your problem?

In our study, Penny Liberatos and I noticed that, of the 6 breast characteristics suggested by the Huggins study, 4 were most prevalent: lack of breast changes in pregnancy, lack of breast changes postpartum, wide spacing, and asymmetry. While stretch marks were a popular characteristic, in my clinical experience, the presence or absence of them on breasts that were otherwise developed does not seem to be related to milk output—but stretch marks on very underdeveloped breasts do raise my suspicions. Because the majority of our study respondents had a high BMI, it also seemed impractical to consider breast shape; it is possible for a woman to have large, full breasts but still have IGT. Indeed, because there is so much fat tissue in these breasts, IGT is very often missed in these women—appearance alone can't tell the whole story of what is or isn't there.

Another important aspect of a mother's history is whether she had to offer a supplement to her baby within the first two days of his birth. In this time frame, a baby only needs a very small amount of colostrum—1/4 teaspoon in a 20-minute feeding session is normal transfer for a newborn. There are women who believe they didn't make any colostrum, but this is highly unlikely, since the hormonal setting of pregnancy and the immediate postpartum (when colostrum is made) is so drastically different from the hormonal setting of normal lactation. Also, the very small amount of colostrum that is needed can be made by the glandular tissue that is there, and storage capacity—how much milk a mother can accumulate and store between feedings—isn't of consequence when we're dealing with such small amounts.

There is a good reason why some babies don't wet or soil diapers in those first 48 hours, though: they might be unable to transfer the colostrum that's there. This can happen for a variety of reasons, but the most common are oral irregularities (such as tongue tie) in the baby or incorrect positioning/latching. If these issues are not immediately noticed and resolved, they could cause or further complicate very early breastfeeding problems. However, low milk output due to IGT does not typically reveal itself during a regular (short) postpartum hospital stay.

Low milk supply that starts later, say after the 4- or 5-week mark, is also not likely to be caused by IGT, but it could be if those 4 weeks were spent with the baby barely hanging on to his growth curve. A "vanishing milk supply" is more likely due to...you guessed it, a tongue-tied or otherwise unable to effectively transfer milk infant.

The following decision tree can help you determine whether your lactation insufficiency might have been caused by IGT, something else, or more than one factor.

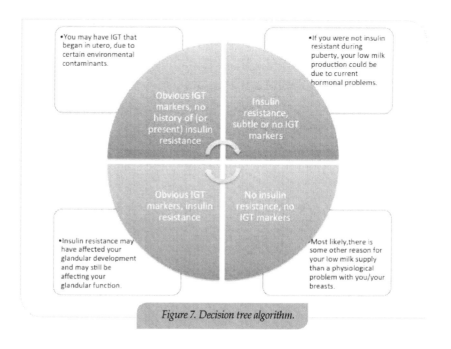

Figure 7. Decision tree algorithm.

As you can see, there may always be some uncertainty about exactly why you aren't (or weren't, if your breastfeeding days are behind you already) able to make a full milk supply.

There are so many variables that can affect lactation, and definitive identification of which of those affected yours can be difficult to pin down.

You may not ever truly know whether your issue was IGT, sufficient glandular tissue that simply didn't respond to the hormones of pregnancy and lactation, a complicated birth/postpartum period that compromised breastfeeding management during a critical window, or something to do with your baby's ability to adequately transfer milk. You can know, though, that regardless of the reason(s) breastfeeding didn't work as you hoped it would, you are still your baby's mother, and your love for that child isn't measured in drops, milliliters, or ounces of milk.

> For me it's possible with the help of herbs, drinks, and certain foods for me and infant formula for my son. For some women breastfeeding isn't possible. The most important thing to remember is that it doesn't matter if you breastfeed or bottle-feed. What matters is that we show our children that we love them and will always be there for them. Love matters most.

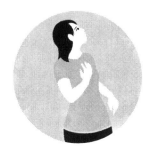

Chapter 4

Glandular Development, BMI, and Insulin

T he following is a simplification of the hormonal processes that drive breast development—what actually occurs is far more complex. While the scientific literature and clinical observations provide insight into why or how some women experience insufficient glandular development, we haven't yet arrived at a conclusive, definite factor or factors that affect most women who are exposed to them or that most women with lactation failure have in common.

Emerging research has offered insight into the roles of insulin and insulin-like growth factor 1 (IGF1) in the development of the mammary gland. I do not discuss this intricate, complex endocrine sequence in this book other than to relate it to the more obvious consequence (or cause?) of insulin dysregulation: overweight or obesity (high BMI).

It is important to note that glandular development of the breasts is known to occur during three key periods in a female's life: during her development in utero (before she is born), during puberty, and during pregnancy. For a more detailed description of the biochemistry of the glandular development of the breast, please refer to Lawrence and Lawrence (2011) and Macias and Hinck (2012), which provided the basis for this chapter.

Breast Development

There are three periods in the life of a human female during which her breasts develop: the embryonic period, when she is in her mother's womb; the pubertal period, during her adolescent years; and during pregnancy, when the hormones of pregnancy finalize the breasts' preparations for making milk (Lawrence & Lawrence, 2011). Abnormal development during the embryonic and/or pubertal periods may be responsible for little or no breast changes during pregnancy, the hormonal milieu at the time of the woman's conception could be to blame—or both could be factors.

In their book, *The Breastfeeding Mother's Guide to Making More Milk,* West and Marasco cited literature (Fenton, Hamm, Birnbaum, & Youngblood, 2002; Gladen & Rogan, 1995; Guillette et al., 2006; Markey, Rubin, Soto, & Sonnenschein, 2003) that suggests that exposure to certain chemicals and their endocrine-disrupting properties may cause the breasts to not properly develop during the embryonic stage.

These environmental exposures of the mother may have consequences for the mammary gland development of the child she is carrying. Markey et al. reported that the effects of bisphenol A, which mimics estrogen and disrupts processes that are reliant upon a specific level of estrogen in the body, may be a cause for compromised mammary gland development in populations that are exposed to high levels of the chemical.

Fenton et al. (2002) reported stunted glandular development in rat breasts upon gestational exposure to 2,3,7,8-tetrocholordibenzo-p-dioxin (TCDD). Gladen and Rogan (1995) suggested that exposure to dichlorodiphenyl dichloroethene (DDE), a by-product of the pesticide DDT, in a Mexican agricultural valley may have affected lactation capabilities in that population. Their hypothesis, however, was based only on the presence of DDE exposure and a higher occurrence of lactation failure among the women living in that valley. No measures correlating the levels of exposure with the severity of hypoplasia or to correlate the degree of lactation dysfunction were reported.

Guillette et al. (2006) reported that 18.5% of girls in a similar Mexican valley village to that studied by Gladen and Rogan (1995) had no palpable glandular tissue, but adipose (fat) tissue was present. The breasts appeared to be of an appropriate size compared to the rest of the girls' bodies but were lacking in glandular tissue. This is similar to current clinical observations of "big enough" breasts that mysteriously don't make enough milk.

A more recent review of studies supported the hypothesis that exposure in utero or during early life to endocrine-disrupting environmental contaminants may have an adverse effect on mammary gland development, which could possibly affect women's lactation capability and their susceptibility to cancer of the breast (Rudel, Fenton, Ackerman, Euling, & Makris, 2011).

Dioxins, in particular, have been found to have endocrine-disrupting effects on humans. A known endocrine (hormone) disruptor, dioxin can block the action of estrogen in the body, change the number of estrogen receptor sites, alter the rate of production of hormones in the body, replace hormones on carrier proteins in the bloodstream, and cause adverse health effects (some barely noticeable, others very severe) by making some or all of the naturally occurring hormones in the body unavailable for use (Moore, 2007). This effect of dioxin can cause an interruption of mammary gland development and differentiation (Vorderstrasse, Fenton, Bohn, Cundiff, & Lawrence, 2004).

It is important to consider, however, that these chemicals are rather ubiquitous in our modern times. We are all exposed to them to some degree. It would logically follow, then, that a larger number of readily visible conditions, such as incomplete breast development, would be seen if our population load were as heavy as it ought to be given how widespread these chemicals are.

On the other hand, many of the mothers who are giving birth today may have been conceived not long after 1987, which is when the United States implemented more stringent controls on the industrial emissions of dioxins (U.S. Environmental Protection Agency, 2011). The level of dioxins in the environment has decreased by 90% since these controls were put in place, so it will be interesting to see whether the generation of girls who were conceived around the turn of the century is as affected as those born in the late 1980s and early 1990s. For additional discussion about the potential role of dioxins in insufficient glandular development, visit my blog *(http://dianaibclc.com/2012/02/28/if-breastfeeding-is-normal-lets-clean-up-the-environment/).*

In clinical observation, I've seen cases of IGT that I might guess (and we really have no way to conclusively verify which breasts were compromised in utero and which were affected by problems in puberty, though other aspects of a woman's health history might give us clues) were "programmed" before the women were born—something interrupted the regular process of cell differentiation while they were tiny embryos. These are women who lower their nursing tank during a lactation consult to reveal dramatically hypoplastic-appearing breasts but who report absolutely no other evidence of hormonal irregularities. These are breasts we might call *"mosquito-bite breasts"* because they are so tiny, or the woman might have a chest that looks more like a man's. These are also the breasts that have "phantom" stretch marks—stretch marks where there was obviously no rapid growth. This is the "classic" presentation of IGT.

In my practice and experience, only a very small percentage of women with IGT fall into this category. In our study, Penny Liberatos and I asked whether respondents or their mothers might have lived in communities where there might have been a higher level of exposure to environmental contaminants, such as an agricultural area or near a paper mill. Around 25% of mothers with IGT markers (widely spaced breasts, asymmetry, and little or no breast changes in pregnancy or postpartum) responded that they believed they lived in communities where exposure to environmental toxins was high. Close to 30% believed that their mothers did. It's important to note, however, that, for both questions, the majority of respondents answered, "I don't know," so this rate may actually be higher.

Research into the numbers of mothers without breastfeeding difficulties who report these same beliefs is necessary in order to have a true basis for comparison. If around 30% of all women share this background, this rate among the mothers with IGT characteristics doesn't really tell us anything. For now, it's a high enough rate to warrant further attention and questioning.

> *I'm frequently asked whether IGT might have happened because of exposure to cigarette smoke, either in utero (the woman's mother smoked while she was pregnant) family members who smoked in the home, or because the mother, herself, smoked during her teen years. Although cigarettes have been shown to exhibit a high dioxin-like potential (Kasai et al., 2006), it is unlikely that exposure to cigarette smoke alone could have the profound effects on glandular development that are seen in women with lactation insufficiency. If exposure to cigarette smoke were capable of such damage, we might see a higher geographic distribution of IGT in areas of the country where smoking is less regulated (for example, where it is still permitted in restaurants and other indoor venues) and more widely practiced, but that doesn't seem to be the case from clinical observations and the data we collected in our study.*

In the majority of cases of breasts that appear to have not developed fully, there seems to be some other endocrinopathy. Something either subtle or very obvious was or continues to be "off" in the mother's regular hormonal processes. In the rest of this chapter, I examine the primary hormones that are involved in glandular development and function and share the research to date on what we suspect or can conclude about the effects of these hormonal issues.

In this book, I do not seek to address lactation failure that is caused by preglandular irregularities—hormonal problems in women whose breasts are fully and adequately developed. For more information about those milk-making issues, please refer to *The Breastfeeding Mother's Guide to Making More Milk* (West & Marasco, 2008). Also, remember that your breastfeeding difficulties may be attributable to both glandular and preglandular (and even postglandular) factors. Some of the hormonal "misfires" that are described in this chapter could affect both glandular development and the ability of what glandular tissue is there to perform to its maximum milk-making potential.

Although in this book I also do not seek to prescribe or recommend courses of action to rectify or treat endocrine irregularities, the understanding that you will hopefully gain from this chapter might offer some insight into what your individual milk-making problems might be so that you can have an informed conversation with your health care provider (or identify a physician or other practitioner who can help you). I see far too many mothers run to purchase the latest herb or medication because it worked for her "boob twin," or another mother with low milk supply. After reading this chapter, you will be better equipped to narrow down and explore what happened along the way with *your* glandular development and what approach you might take to address those issues.

Progesterone

The role of progesterone in breast development is well understood. During adolescence, after a girl begins having menstrual cycles, both estrogen and progesterone act on breast development. Estrogen is responsible for the growth of fatty tissue in the breast, and progesterone stimulates the development of the glandular tissue that will characterize the "milk factory" later in life.[1]

---

1   Remember that estrogen and progesterone are the lead characters in this story but that other hormones are involved in pubertal and pregnancy-related glandular development.

Development of the Parenchyma

In anatomical terms, the functional part of the breast, the milk factory, is called the *parenchyma*. The parenchyma needs the fatty tissue, or the "cosmetically pleasing" part of the breast, to be present around it, so that it has a place to anchor itself. Imagine that the estrogen-fed fatty tissue is a vast harbor and the progesterone-fed parenchyma are the ships and boats, sailing into the harbor and putting down moorings, month by month, cycle by cycle.

Obviously, if a girl is not experiencing regular periods at the time that her breasts require estrogen (to expand the capacity of the harbor) and progesterone (to attract more vessels to moor there), there may be a problem with lactation in the future.

Corpus Luteum

In simple terms, the first half of the menstrual cycle is considered the follicular, or ovulatory, phase. There are lots of hormones in this ovulatory-phase ensemble cast, but let's call estrogen the star. Once ovulation takes place, there are other hormones that play supporting roles, but the star of this second phase of the menstrual cycle, the luteal phase (named after our friend, the corpus luteum), is progesterone.

Amenorrhea (or lack of menstrual periods) for any reason—an eating disorder, elite athleticism, or hormonal disturbances such as PCOS that limit (or prohibit entirely) the number of ovulatory cycles a young woman has—can reduce that sustained, cyclical exposure to estrogen and progesterone that her breasts must have in order to develop properly.

What sometimes occurs is that estrogen keeps the stage; without ovulation, progesterone never upstages estrogen for the lead role during that second half of the month/cycle. This unopposed exposure to estrogen does not promote good health and, over time, may be a risk factor for additional problems, such as cancer or endometriosis.

A teen with PCOS may have periods, but if she is not ovulating, progesterone may be insufficient to promote glandular development in adolescence. This is because, as a woman ovulates, a spot is left on her ovary. It is called the *corpus luteum,* or "yellow body," and it secretes progesterone. If she does not become pregnant after ovulation, the corpus luteum will send out the progesterone for, ideally, 12–14 days. When it stops doing so, the rich lining that had been built in the uterus is shed, and the woman gets her period. Spotting before her period or luteal phases of less than 12 days may indicate a problem with the body's ability to maintain the appropriate level of progesterone at given times.

This is a key point for mothers with insufficient breast development who also experience recurrent miscarriages that are attributable to low progesterone. For whatever reason, the corpora lutea in these women don't put out enough progesterone, or the progesterone that is put out is unable to do its job (perhaps also in breast development?) because other hormones are getting in the way. Brannian, Zhao, and McElroy (1999) suggested that perhaps leptin, a hormone secreted by fat cells, blocks the action of insulin and restricts the ability of the ovaries to secrete sufficient progesterone. This may be a mechanism by which a BMI greater than 25 can influence glandular development and, as a result, milk production.

Progesterone and Pregnancy

When a woman becomes pregnant, the corpus luteum receives a signal from the implanted embryo to continue sending out progesterone. This allows the built-up uterine lining to remain intact while the embryo makes himself at home and some of his cells become his placenta. At around the 6-week mark of pregnancy (4 weeks after fertilization), the corpus luteum ceases to sustain the pregnancy with progesterone. The placenta has, if all has gone well, taken over this important job at this point. Typically, progesterone levels during pregnancy (thanks to the placenta) can be 300 times greater than they are at other times when the woman is not pregnant.

Even when a pregnancy "sticks," with a placenta that secretes enough progesterone to see the pregnancy to term, progesterone can still be a culprit in lack of breast development during pregnancy and, ultimately, in the inability to produce enough milk to exclusively breastfeed. There may be a minimum level of progesterone that is needed to keep a pregnancy viable that is lower than what is needed to trigger the formation and development of the breast alveoli during pregnancy. These alveoli are all-important pieces of the milk factory for many reasons. One reason is that, inside them, prolactin-receptor sites are formed in response to breast stimulation in the early postpartum days. If prolactin levels aren't able to spike high enough (because of baby's inability to adequately stimulate the breasts or because some other hormonal action that should not be taking place is preventing the secretion of enough prolactin), fewer prolactin receptors will be formed in the breast alveoli; this may result in long-term difficulty making milk. Similarly, if the secretion of progesterone in pregnancy isn't robust enough to stimulate the development and growth of enough alveoli, there won't be enough places for those prolactin receptors to appear. Additionally, the alveoli are where milk is secreted and stored. It makes sense that if there are not enough of these places where milk is made and kept, less milk will be produced.

Another possible progesterone issue could be that not enough progesterone-fed development took place during adolescence. The hormones of pregnancy may be adequate, but there's nowhere for them to go. To put it another way, in this case, you might have a few smart, good throwers on your football team, but if there aren't enough players on the field to catch the ball, fewer touchdowns will be scored. Mothers who seek to improve their ability to make milk for another baby after a difficult breastfeeding experience may be very interested in trying progesterone supplements to help develop more glandular tissue in pregnancy, when the body would normally already be working on this.

There is one case report (Bodley & Powers, 1999) of a mother who used progesterone supplements during the early part of her second pregnancy and experienced a dramatic increase in her milk output for that baby over what she was able to do for her first. While this does offer a consideration for mothers with IGT, it is important to realize that repeated pregnancies (and exposure to pregnancy hormones—remember that pregnancy progesterone levels can be 300 times greater than nonpregnant levels and are sustained for several months when the pregnancy is carried to term) may, without additional intervention, act on the breasts and increase their milk-making capability, especially if other hormonal issues (such as those associated with high BMI) are resolved before that pregnancy begins.

Clinical experience tells us this is true even of mothers with no trouble with milk production. Many have reported having more milk with subsequent babies than they had for their first. The case report of Bodley and Powers (1999) shares the experience of a mother in her fifth pregnancy, however. She had one miscarriage before her first child was born and two before her second child was born. She was diagnosed with luteal phase defect, and progesterone was most definitely an issue for this mother. Progesterone in early pregnancy may be an option for you but only if your breast development was stunted by insufficient progesterone and only if there are enough "receivers on your football team."

Insulin Resistance and Progesterone

It is also important to consider that if progesterone is not your problem and insulin resistance is actually to blame for your milk-production troubles (more likely), adding progesterone may, in fact, exacerbate the problem you're seeking to solve. Wada et al. (2010) studied the effect of progesterone on blood sugar and insulin signaling and had this to say:

> Epidemiological studies have revealed that administration of progestin for contraceptive usage is associated with increased incidence of type 2 diabetes. A hyperglycemic

hyperinsulinemic clamp study showed that progesterone administration for 8 weeks reduced whole body glucose uptake in humans. Concerning the role of progesterone in insulin secretion, female progesterone receptor knockout mice demonstrated a reduced fasting blood glucose level with elevation of serum insulin by increased β-cell proliferation, indicating the possible relation of progesterone with β-cell proliferation and/or function. However, the precise mechanism by which progesterone causes insulin resistance is so far unknown. (p. E887)

This gives us reason to pause and remember that what works to improve milk production in one mother not might not work in another. Indeed, the wrong approach can even make milk production more difficult. Learn as much as you can about your body before running for the latest cream or suppository that worked for a mother who might be your "boob twin" with similar physical features. Without knowing what is going on hormonally, your efforts could set you back more than they help you.

Some outstanding research into progesterone levels in pregnancy has been done by Dr. Thomas Hilgers with the Pope Paul VI Institute in Omaha, Nebraska. Dr. Hilgers produced, on the basis of research about progesterone and optimal gestational outcomes, the following chart, which may be used, in cooperation with your physician, to monitor whether your progesterone levels in pregnancy are, in fact, optimal or whether your placenta is enabling you to just get by. If you believe that progesterone is a significant contributor to your mammary hypoplasia, *The Medical and Surgical Practice of NaPro-*

Technology, by Dr. Hilgers, may offer you additional insight. It is available for order at *http://naprotechnology.com/naprotext.htm.*

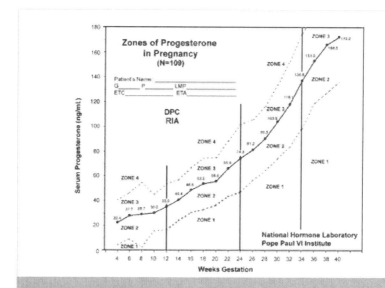

Figure 8. From Hilgers (2014). The Medical and Surgical Practice of NaProTechnology (p. 731)
© 2014 by Pope Paul VI Institute for the Study of Human Reproduction.
All rights reserved. Retrieved from http://www.naprotechnology.com/progesterone.htm.
Reprinted with permission.

Charting Fertility Signs

The endocrine system is very complex. A woman can gain great insight into her body and learn a lot about how her cycles are working by charting her monthly fertility signs. There are many resources available for learning how to recognize and monitor your basal body temperature (your temperature when you first wake up, before you move or get out of bed), cervical fluid (which changes in response to various hormones at different times in your cycle and offers information about what's happening hormonally in your body on any given day), and cervical texture and position (whether your cervix is high or low and soft or firm; these are clues to your hormonal state and where you are in your cycle.).

You may think you have a "normal" menstrual cycle, but are you ovulating at least 12 days before your period starts (ideally, 14–15 days before)? Do you ovulate at the same time every month, or are your cycles irregular? Are your basal body temperatures significantly higher after you've ovulated (because the hormones of the ovulatory phase suppress this temperature and progesterone slightly raises it), or is your body showing a lesser response?

My favorite resource is Toni Weschler's (2006) *Taking Charge of Your Fertility*. Yes, fertility awareness, as this method of understanding and monitoring your cyclic hormonal signs is sometimes called, can be used to achieve or prevent pregnancy. It can also be a noninvasive, reliable method of figuring out what's going on hormonally that might affect what is referred to as *the reproductive axis*. This term represents the interplay between the hypothalamus and pituitary (both are glands in your brain) and the ovaries.

If, after charting a few cycles, you notice very slight or no signif-icant increase in your basal body temperature after your cervical fluid has dried up (an indication that you've ovulated), if you have spotting before your period (it's much easier to tell this is happening regularly if you're keeping a record of it!), or if the number of days between ovulation and the start of your period is less than 12, you will have specific data, information about *your* body, to bring to your physician, and an indisputable basis for the concerns you are raising about your progesterone levels.

Many doctors are understandably reluctant to prescribe or test for conditions they might not be aware of or they might not suspect you have. A comprehensive understanding of how your body should be working, coupled with symptoms that it might not be, can give you a solid foundation for a confident, empowered discussion with a medical professional about how to obtain more information (for example, by blood tests or ultrasound) and which avenues you can pursue together to achieve better results.

Can a Higher BMI Affect Lactation?

This question has been studied, and the answer is yes—maternal overweight has been identified as a potential risk factor for the delayed onset of lactation (Chapman & Pérez-Escamilla, 1999), which can generate a snowball effect of early supplementation and poor breastfeeding management in those critical early hours and days. However, we are reminded that obesity or overweight do not always predict lactation difficulty. Many women with a high BMI go on to produce plenty of milk, even overproduce in some cases, and not all women with milk-production issues have a BMI over 30, though it seems that a growing percentage does. The scientific literature also suggests overweight or obesity during adolescence can affect pubertal development (Burt Solorzano & McCartney, 2010).

In our study of mothers with low milk supply, just over 60% of respondents with IGT markers reported being overweight or obese during adolescence. This represents a percentage much higher than the estimated percentage (33.2%) of U.S. children aged 6–19 who are considered to be overweight or obese (Ogden, Carroll, Kit, & Flegal, 2012). The difference would be even greater if we were comparing a population that more closely approximated our study population, primarily white females. More research is needed to explore the possible relationship between adolescent BMI or perhaps adolescent diet and mammary gland development.

Related (though more research is necessary to conclude how closely) to BMI is the diet that is consumed during adolescence. Today's new mothers grew up during what I call the "Snackwell's era," referring to a popular brand of snacks that were, as dietary recommendations of that time encouraged, processed to be low in fat. In order to be appealing, however, these products had way more sugar than their regular-fat counterparts (perhaps they still do; there are many low-fat products still marketed as "healthy" foods, even though current science suggests that dietary fat doesn't cause body fat; instead, more sugar and simple carbohydrates do). A relevant study of rabbits examined the role of adolescent diet on mammary gland development during midpregnancy (Hue-Beauvais et al., 2011). These researchers fed an obesogenic diet (high fat, high sugar) to prepubertal rabbits, then compared the rabbits' mammary gland development at mid-pregnancy to that of rabbits fed a control diet. What they found was that the rabbits fed the high-sugar diet had more rapid pubertal breast development but lower capacity for lactation after the glandular development of pregnancy.

If these findings were to be replicated in longitudinal human studies and, thereby, implicate adolescent diet in future lactation insufficiency, the impact on U.S. food policy would be profound. This type of research, which measures nutritional status and dietary intake in prepubertal girls and then follows them into adulthood and examines such outcomes as weight status, reproductive axis functioning, and lactation, is sorely needed. For now, we can look to our rabbit friends for possibilities of what is going wrong for us.

> *The discussion of risk factors for lactation insufficiency in this chapter includes extensive reference to BMI. Although it offers researchers a frame of reference for measuring and categorizing weight status, BMI alone is not a measure or categorization of overall health or wellness. Just as an individual can have a high BMI but be very muscular and physically fit with no risk factors for disease or mortality, many women with a high pre-pregnant BMI go on to lactate and breastfeed without incident or issue. An intelligent discussion of BMI was recently presented by Jane Brody (2014) in the New York Times (http://well.blogs.nytimes. com/2014/04/14/a-number-that-may-not-add-up/).*

Rasmussen, Hilson, and Kjolhede (2001) reported a connection between a BMI greater than 30 and impaired/delayed lactogenesis II (the production of copious milk). Nommsen-Rivers, Chantry, Peerson, Cohen, and Dewey (2010) published another study whose findings supported a BMI over 30 as a cause for delayed lactogenesis II in first-time mothers. However, maternal edema created the same effect when it was used in their statistical model.

In discussions among clinicians, there are different opinions about why this relationship between a BMI of greater than 30 and a shortened time of breastfeeding might happen. Is it because of incorrect, hurtful expectations about those of us who are overweight, that perhaps we don't care about what is best for our health and the health of our children? Or is it because breastfeeding with large, pendulous breasts presents practical, mechanical challenges not faced by mothers with different body types? These factors may contribute to the observed shorter breastfeeding duration among mothers with a high prepregnancy BMI, but there is little question that some aspect of the altered physiology when weight is not normal is necessary for successful lactation. Does obesity cause this problem, or does the problem cause obesity (and later, lactation difficulty)? If we take the view that impaired lactation is a *symptom* of *something else* about our bodies maybe out of whack, we can approach the problem more holistically, with the aim of improving overall health, not just milk production.

Another consideration with regard to higher BMI and lactation is the possible reduced effect of infant suckling on prolactin levels in the early days postpartum. Ostrum and Ferris (1993) found lower prolactin levels in mothers with insulin-dependent diabetes. These findings suggest that additional care should be taken to ensure that these mothers have good control over their blood sugar and are feeding their babies or stimulating their breasts appropriately and frequently. This is, of course, good guidance for all new breast-feeding mothers, but it is of special importance for mothers with diabetes (who may or may not have a BMI over 30; it is the insulin dependence that seems significant here).

Rasmussen and Kjolhede (2004) found that prolactin levels in women who had a BMI of greater than 26 did not go as high after their babies fed as they did in mothers who were of normal weight before they got pregnant. Going back to what we know about prolactin-receptor theory and the importance of those early, frequent prolactin spikes, it's possible that the lower prolactin levels (and spikes that don't go as high) could lead to fewer receptor sites being created in those early days; this could reduce a mother's ultimate milk-making potential.

In this study, the response of prolactin levels to suckling at day 7 postpartum was similar in high-BMI and normal-BMI mothers, so this effect only occurred in the very beginning, but by day 7, babies that are not thriving and gaining weight are already being frantically supplemented, often without anyone making sure that their mothers' breasts are being adequately and regularly stimulated. Additional, valuable time in that prolactin-receptor window may be lost before anyone thinks to address the lactation issue while also addressing the feed-the-baby priority. This study only included 17 mothers in their group of women with BMIs of greater than 26. It is difficult to draw conclusions based on a sample this small, but perhaps we have some clues to guide further research.

Insulin

Through the observation and study of over 1,000 mothers with lactation insufficiency and a review of the available literature about glandular development and lactation, it has become evident to me that the hormone insulin is a key player in this drama.

The work of Marasco et al. (2000) and West and Marasco (2008) has already informed the lactation support community of practitioners about the relationship between PCOS and breastfeeding problems, and—insulin resistance is part of that syndrome.

According to the U.S. Department of Health and Human Services, National Institutes of Health (NIH; 2013), poly-cystic ovarian syndrome (PCOS), also and formerly called Stein-Leventhal syndrome, affects at least five million women in the United States alone. Symptoms may include weight gain, acne, scalp hair loss, hirsutism (excessive body hair where hair does not characteristi-cally grow), irregular or absent menstrual periods, infertility, and ovarian cysts. In addition, those with PCOS are more likely to be insulin resistant, which, if not addressed and treated, may lead to the development of diabetes and cardiovascular disease. Obesity exacerbates the symptoms of PCOS, but where insulin resistance is present, weight loss can be more difficult. Diagnosis of PCOS can be tricky because it requires the presence of two of three criteria or all three: excess of androgen hormones (such as testosterone and DHEA); irregular or no ovulation, which can be caused by a variety of hormonal dysfunctions; and polycystic ovaries. Because a woman can have PCOS without actually having polycystic ovaries, the NIH is calling for experts to change the name of the syndrome because its current name may delay or inhibit proper diagnosis and treatment. A name that is better descriptive of the complex web of metabolic, hypothalamic, pituitary, ovarian, and adrenal functions that occur in patients with the syndrome will advance its study and the health of women and their children. Understanding that women seek help from various health care providers for their symptoms of PCOS is key to improving their care. Women with lactation problems that are not solved by correcting breastfeeding management or oral anomalies (such as tongue tie) in the infant should be evaluated for insulin resistance and androgen excess, regardless of ovarian function or fertility history.

The Role of Insulin Resistance

Insulin resistance, which precedes type 2 diabetes and is a symptom of metabolic syndrome, is a condition in which the body uses insulin (to regulate blood sugar) less effectively.

More and more insulin is needed to regulate blood sugar, until, if it is not resolved, the body stops being able to produce enough insulin to keep blood sugar levels in a normal range (diabetes). A person might have insulin resistance for years before ever developing diabetes and have no idea they have it. Insulin resistance is not a condition with obvious symptoms.

A recent, groundbreaking study revealed that when a mother is insulin resistant, a particular gene is expressed more prominently than in insulin-sensitive individuals. This genetic expression confirmed the relationship between insulin resistance and insufficient milk supply (Lemay et al., 2013).

This information correlates well with what Dr. Liberatos and I learned about our study population of mothers with lactation insufficiency: that a greater percentage of our respondents reported a prepregnant BMI that could be classified as overweight (BMI= 25.0–29.9) or obese (BMI 30 or greater) compared to what is found among the general population.

While not always comorbid—an individual can be insulin resistant and appear lean and thin, just as a person with a higher BMI may be appropriately insulin sensitive and healthy—insulin resistance and high BMI are often seen together.

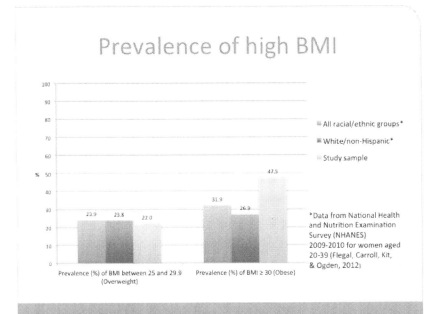

Figure 9. The data in this graphic represent an interim analysis of approximately 1,000 respondents. A preliminary analysis of the complete data set from the study did not indicate a significant deviation from this representation.

These rates of pre-pregnant BMI ranges of greater than 25 and 30 and greater were remarkable when compared to the general population, and this supported the suggestions of other studies that the hormonal state inherent in obesity may be related to lactation dysfunction—but does a BMI of greater than 30 impair the ability of the existing glandular tissue to lactate properly, or is insulin resistance during puberty to blame for inadequate and incomplete development of the breast glands?

It is obvious that we are dealing with a very complex web of interdependent factors. One piece of the puzzle, which is related to high BMI, may be leptin, a hormone that is secreted by fat cells. Its short-term purpose is to regulate appetite and its long-term purpose is to regulate body weight. Brannian, Zhao, and McElroy (1999) also found that leptin may limit or inhibit the production of progesterone by the ovaries but only when insulin was also present. If we think about what we know to be true about progesterone and glandular development, it makes sense that excess leptin *plus* excess insulin might result in insufficient progesterone each month to stimulate glandular growth of the breasts, even if ovulation and regular menstrual cycles are occurring.

Insulin resistance is prevalent in Western societies and often goes unrecognized until type 2 diabetes emerges. In many people with insulin resistance, there are no outward symptoms. Some may have a condition called *acanthosis nigricans,* which is a darkening of skin either around the neck or in patches in places such as the elbows, knees, knuckles, and armpits. Just over a decade ago, the means to assess for insulin resistance was complicated and difficult, requiring repeated blood samples over a period of a few hours to measure blood glucose, insulin, or both. A simple explanation of this procedure, called hyperglycemic (high blood sugar), hyper-insulinemic (high insulin), or euglycemic (normal blood sugar) glucose clamps, can be found at this link: *http://www.diabeteshealth. com/read/2007/11/06/5500/whats-a-glucose-clamp-anyway/.*

Although glucose clamp techniques are the gold standard and the only way to assess *exactly* how insulin is being secreted and used in an individual's body, recent and ongoing research has revealed simpler techniques for assessing insulin sensitivity in people with normal blood sugar—people who *don't yet have recurrent fasting blood glucose (sugar) levels in the diabetic or prediabetic ranges* (over 120 mg/

dL or over 100 mg/dL, respectively). *Those under the care of a health care provider for problems with insulin sensitivity may have more precise results with a different mathematical assessment than what follows for those who are normoglycemic.* Also, those individuals with known problems with glucose metabolism (high or low blood sugar) are almost definitely insulin resistant. Diabetes is the end state of insulin resistance when it is allowed to continue.

All of these techniques for assessing insulin sensitivity use variables that should be easy to test for in a routine fasting blood test; these include triglyceride, insulin, and glucose levels as well as easily obtained values, such as waist circumference and BMI. Assessments that have been compared to the euglycemic clamp technique include:

- Fasting insulin level

- Homeostasis model assessment (HOMA)

- Insulin-to-glucose ratio

- Bennett index

- McAuley index

The McAuley index (McAuley et al., 2001) was shown in studies to be the most effective in correctly diagnosing insulin resistance in *normoglycemic individuals* without missing cases or offering false positives. If your blood glucose is not normal, you may wish to consult your health care provider for assistance with another assessment of your insulin sensitivity (although your abnormal blood sugars are already suggestive of insulin resistance). The McAuley et al. article comprehensively explains which indices are available and under which circumstances each is best applied. The McAuley index is a mathematical formula that uses fasting insulin (measured in micro International Units per milliliter [μIU/mL] or milliunits per liter [mu/L]) and triglycerides (measured in millimoles per liter [mmol/L] or converted from milligrams per deciliter [mg/dL] with a calculator such as the one found at *http://www.onlineconversion.com/cholesterol.htm*).

The formula is as follows:

Insulin Sensitivity Index = exp[2.63 – 0.28 ln(insulin) – 0.31 ln(triglycerides)]

A value under 5.8 is considered to indicate insulin resistance. For example, in an individual with a triglyceride value of 145 mg/dL (this is converted to mmol/L, and this value is used, in this case, 1.6370) and a fasting insulin of 15.8 μIU/mL, the following calculation (if you have a smartphone with a calculator, the advanced logarithmic function buttons are revealed when you hold your phone in landscape mode) would be made:

ISI = exp(2.63 – 0.28 ln 15.8 – 0.31 ln 1.6370)

ISI = exp(2.63 – 0.7728 – 0.1528)

ISI = exp(1.7044)

ISI = 5.498

This patient should be advised that she may be insulin resistant, even if her blood glucose is normal. Measures to improve her health, such as a higher protein diet and physical activity, or prescription medication, may be advised.

Another patient may have a fasting triglyceride value of 34 mg/ dL (this value is converted to 0.3839 mmol/L) and an insulin value of 9.0. Her insulin sensitivity index would be calculated as follows:

ISI = exp(2.63 − 0.28 ln 9.0 − 0.31 ln 0.3839)

ISI = exp(2.63 − 0.6152 − 0.2968)

ISI = exp(2.3116)

ISI = 10.091

This patient is probably not insulin resistant.

So, Does Insulin Resistance Prevent Me from Making Milk? Can I Still Have IGT?

This is a complicated question, and another area where more research is definitely needed because there are insulin-resistant women who make plenty of milk (perhaps their pubertal breast development was robust?) and a confirmed relationship between insulin resistance and low milk output. We do know that insulin is important. Insulin has a direct action on the mammary gland during breast development and is vital to the production and secretion of colostrum (lactogenesis I), in lactogenesis II (when lots of milk arrives after the placenta is born, usually around 2 or 3 days postpartum), and continued lactation.

Berlato and Doppler (2009) examined the action of insulin and insulin-like growth factors on mammary gland development and the ability of those cells to secrete milk in mice. They found that particular cells in the breast must remain insulin sensitive to develop properly and function in the presence of other hormones of lactation. While this doesn't address insulin and glandular development directly, it does provide some insight into why we might be seeing so much insulin resistance among mothers with full but perhaps slightly hypoplastic-appearing breasts. It provides some support for what we know to be true about herbs and supplements that seem to help with milk production: they enhance blood sugar metabolism and insulin sensitivity.

In addition, while mouse models are valuable for studying the effect of isolated factors (such as hormones or hormone receptors or the effect of one factor on another) on mammary gland development and milk-making ability, it is important to consider that, anatomically, mice are different from humans; their mammary glands alone can represent 5–10% of their total body weight, and they need to produce enough milk to feed 8–12 babies at once! Despite these limitations, though, mouse models offer some important clues to what might be going on in humans.

Another mouse model that offers some insight was presented by Sun, Shushanov, LeRoith, and Wood (2011). These researchers found that when receptors for insulin-like growth factor were decreased (such as, perhaps, when there was too much insulin-like growth factor circulating during adolescent breast development), the body adapted by making fewer receptors, resulting in fewer alveoli (milk-making sites in the breast). However, in these mice, this did not seem to have a significant effect on whether the mouse pups gained sufficient weight (which was how they measured sufficient milk output in the mice). The study did not account for whether the baby mice fed more frequently or whether the dam's (mamma mouse's) milk was somehow adapted to give her pups a better chance at survival.

What Can I Do If I'm Insulin Resistant?

The problem most of us who've struggled with insulin resistance know all too well is that losing weight helps us normalize insulin sensitivity. However, insulin resistance makes losing weight a more challenging task than it is for those who aren't insulin resistant. It's not as simple as "calories in, calories out," and frustration comes quickly to a person who is eating meticulously (often feeling hungry all the time and fighting sugar cravings) and exercising through a feeling of sheer exhaustion but seeing no results at all.

Those who have been successful losing weight and beating insulin resistance have found that a counted-carbohydrate diet, which is perhaps difficult to get used to at first, can be very effective. Western culture's portions of carbohydrate foods are quite large, much more than we need, and the message that we need "6–11 servings" of whole grains every day is pervasive. If you ever had gestational diabetes, perhaps you were put on a daily eating plan that utilized this strategy to normalize blood sugar and insulin levels until your baby was born: three meals and two or three snacks, with prescribed carbohydrate counts. Usually, meals will have between 30–45 grams of carbohydrates (depending on your current nutritional needs and the severity of your insulin resistance), and snacks will have 15–20 grams. A nutritionist or dietician can help you determine which daily meal plan is best for you.

Paleo Diet

There have been some cases of mothers with low milk production who have moved to a "paleolithic" or "paleo" way of eating and, after a period of time, noticed an improvement in their milk supplies.

The paleo diet emphasizes the consumption of pastured or grass-fed meat, eggs, and lots of sustainably grown vegetables, while minimizing or elminating sugar, soy, processed foods, dairy, and grains, and moderating of fruit intake.

A simple Internet search reveals lots of resources about this dietary lifestyle and testimonials about how it has reversed disease and changed lives. There are other diet plans. Paleo isn't the only one that can provide structure for reducing carbohydrate intake and normalizing insulin sensitivity in your body. Look for ways to eat whole, real foods, and be wary of chemically engineered food-like products, such as artificial sweeteners, which may have fewer calories but often contain ingredients that can have a negative effect on your overall health. A dietician or physician who works with insulin-resistant patients can provide guidance.

The paleo diet, which refers to how our paleolithic ancestors may have eaten, can promote better milk production in mothers who are struggling to exclusively breastfeed. In a study of seven mothers, Mohammad et al. (2009) examined whether a maternal diet of 30% carbohydrates and 55% fat (such as in a paleo-type diet) translated to any change in milk output compared to when the same mothers were fed a diet of 60% carbohydrates and 25% fat (which is closer to the nutrient intake in the standard American diet). While milk output itself was not different enough to be statistically significant, when mothers followed the lower carbohydrate, higher fat (paleo-like) diet, the babies' milk intakes were higher, and they consumed more fat and calories via their mothers' milk. A similar volume of milk had more fat and calories on the lower carbohydrate, higher fat diet. In addition, the mothers had a greater "energy deficit," which would theoretically translate to weight loss, on the lower carbohydrate, higher fat diet. In mothers where insulin sensitivity may be a limiting factor in breast development and function, the adoption of a lower carbohydrate diet that is higher in healthy fats, may improve breastfeeding outcomes and overall health of mother and baby.

Will counting carbs or going paleo definitely increase your milk production? There is some research to suggest that it could (Matsuno, Esrey, Perrault, & Koski, 1999; Mohammad, Sunehag, & Haymond, 2009). Clinical observations indicate that it probably won't hurt your milk supply, and improved health is always a good idea. Whether this way of nourishing your body leads to improved health remains to be seen. There is evidence to support improved overall health on diets that are nothing like the paleo diet. Perhaps different individual physiologies respond to different macronutrient content.

Physical Activity

Along the same lines of good health, daily physical activity is especially vital for those with insulin resistance. You don't have to run a marathon: just 30 minutes each day of walking or other focused movement can help improve your insulin sensitivity and may improve your milk production over time. Even if your milk supply doesn't seem to change, the daily physical activity is indisputably good for your overall health, your mood, and your quality of sleep (even if your baby isn't letting you sleep as much as you used to!) and sets a positive example for your child or children, who want to do everything you do. For strategies about how to begin a daily activity habit while taking care of a baby, check out La Leche League International's *Breastfeeding Today* at *http://viewer. zmags.com/publication/5f3b8aed#/5f3b8aed/6.*

Metformin

Many women with insulin resistance are prescribed metformin to normalize insulin sensitivity and keep blood sugar in a normal range. Some mothers have found that metformin, either through pregnancy, postpartum, or both, has improved their ability to make milk, and this makes a lot of sense, given what we know about insulin and lactation. While anecdotal and clinical experience supports an improvement in milk production for women with insulin resistance who start or resume metformin, Vanky et al. (2012) reported after a randomized, controlled trial that metformin had no effect on breast change/size increase in pregnancy or breastfeeding in women who were obese. However, in this study, metformin was not continued after delivery, and this may (or may not) have been a factor in the outcome. If insulin is an issue for you, discuss your options with your doctor and the potential of these options to help you boost your milk production. Your milk supply troubles may be only a symptom you have that something else is not working properly in your body.

Myo-Inositol

Metformin is not tolerated well by all women. Many stop taking it because the side effect of gastrointestinal distress and diarrhea interferes too much with daily life. There is another option that may be promising for insulin resistant mothers, and it may also improve ovarian function in women with PCOS. Myo-inositol, a naturally occurring substance that our bodies produce, which is also available in foods (as it is a member of the B-complex vitamin group) such as beans, fruits, and nuts, has been shown to have an effect on how our insulin receptors work. It is one ingredient in a supplement that is becoming popular among women with PCOS who wish to become pregnant: Pregnitude (myo-inositol and folic acid).

There have been a few cases of mothers with low milk production trying Pregnitude and seeing an improvement in their milk supplies. Gerli, Papaleo, Ferrari, and DiRenzo (2007) found that myo-inositol helped women with PCOS and a BMI under 37 who were not ovulating to begin ovulating again. The study also noted weight loss among those who were taking the myo-inositol (the experimental dose was 4 grams per day, which is equivalent to eight 500-mg capsules) and weight gain among the placebo group. Another study (Artini et al., 2013) offered similar positive results on ovarian function and an improvement in insulin sensitivity in women with PCOS who were taking myo-inositol (in this study, the dosage was only 2 g per day). Myo-inositol, in very high doses, has also been shown to help with the treatment of obsessive–compulsive disorder and depression (Brink, Viljoen, deKock, Stein, & Harvey, 2004).

It is important to note that myo-inositol has not been *formally studied in pregnancy* but, because of its observed ability to stimulate oxytocin release, may cause *uterine contractions*. The ideal time to see if this supplement might benefit you is *not* when you are pregnant but before you become pregnant. Along those lines, it is decidedly more advisable to improve any insulin issues you may have before you become pregnant. It is wise to find a health care practitioner you trust and discuss options such as myo-inositol with him or her. Often, printing out an abstract to a study (such as those cited in this chapter) and bringing it to your doctor or midwife can prompt her to explore an option that might be new, but beneficial to you.

Preglandular Factors

Glandular lactation failure is too often accompanied by—or perhaps caused by—one or more preglandular and/or postglandular factors. These might be obvious, such as a known thyroid problem, type 2 diabetes, or a long-standing issue with your menstrual cycle or fertility. Preglandular factors that are less obvious might include luteal phase defect and insulin resistance. Lower than optimal progesterone levels during the second half of the menstrual cycle, sometimes resulting in premenstrual spotting, a short luteal phase, or miscarriage, may also represent a preglandular problem with glandular consequences.

Insulin resistance is extremely common in mothers who have what may best be described as a "borderline" hypoplastic breast appearance. Full, perhaps even large breasts with very subtle markers for insufficient glandular development may be considered unremarkable by doctors, nurses, and lactation consultants, even those who are well-trained in breast assessment for breastfeeding. However, with a closer look, asymmetry and wide spacing are often discovered, and palpation of the breasts reveals a paucity of dense glandular tissue in the lower inside quadrants of one or both breasts.

The endocrine system is very complex. Some of the research we have indicates that too much insulin (usually accompanied by a higher than normal BMI) can affect regular processes, such as the menstrual cycle and fertility. Is it really too big a leap to believe that it might have an effect on lactation? Might physiologically driven breastfeeding difficulties be just another symptom of other glitches in the overall system? Understanding your own body and health, asking questions about any medications or behaviors your doctor recommends during your preconception time, and being at a healthy BMI before becoming pregnant can help normalize your hormones. Expert breastfeeding assistance from an IBCLC and the choice of a birth setting that is baby-friendly can help you ensure that your breastfeeding experience gets off to the best start possible.

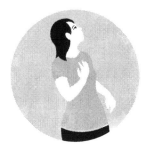

Chapter 5

Feeding Your Baby

New mothers often worry about milk supply. These concerns are so common that they are consistently cited as reasons that mothers wean partially or entirely to breastmilk substitutes (Odom, Li, Scanlon, Perrine, & Grummer-Strawn, 2013). *Perceived insufficient milk* (Neifert & Bunik, 2013) is present when a mother is producing enough milk for her baby, but she believes she is not, perhaps because she incorrectly assigns certain normal behaviors of her baby, such as needing to suckle often or sleeping only when being held, to hunger or dissatisfaction.

There are several factors that can contribute to perceived lactation insufficiency. Sociocultural influences, such as a worried, insistent grandmother who thinks that the baby "just ate" and, therefore, can't possibly need to feed again can undermine a mother's confidence about whether she can satisfy her baby's appetite. Worries that a mother's milk isn't "rich" or "creamy" enough to fatten up a tiny baby are also very common but unfounded. Mismanagement of breastfeeding through a scheduling regime, as is encouraged by popular "baby-training" programs, such as *On Becoming Babywise* (Ezzo & Bucknam, 1995) and *Growing Kids God's Way* (Ezzo & Ezzo, 1993), can wreak havoc on a mother's ability to decipher her baby's cues because she is taught to watch the clock to determine when to feed the baby, not his signals that he is hungry.

Lactation physiology, such as whether a woman believes her breasts are large enough or whether she leaks milk, feels engorged, or experiences a sensation of "let down" when the milk begins to flow, can also affect a mother's perception of her ability to produce milk, even though these feelings *do not predict milk output*.

The woman's psychological state, especially if she is depressed or anxious about her ability to care for her infant, can contribute to perceived lactation insufficiency (Dykes & Williams, 1999). Although an exact prevalence of perceived insufficient milk is difficult to assess, research does indicate a relationship between a perceived "difficult" infant temperament and less understanding of infant cues (McMeekin et al., 2013). A baby who is "fussy" or vocal about his needs may be perceived as hungry, even if he is not, and his mother may conclude that she is unable to produce enough milk for him.

How Can You Know Your Baby Is Getting Enough?

How is a mother to know, then, whether her baby is getting what he needs? While watching diaper output closely is one important way to gauge milk intake, a baby may still wet diapers—or even soil them—while struggling to receive enough calories to grow. Parents may not really know what a wet diaper is supposed to feel like (2–3 tablespoons of water in a clean diaper gives a good estimate) or recognize what properly transitioning stools look like at the end of the first week (there should be no more black, tarry meconium, and the stools should be seedy and yellow–brown).

If a woman suspects that she has this condition, her child should be closely monitored in the hospital, directly after birth for weight loss, wet diapers, and so on. I also think the ob–gyn or hospital nurses that assist with pre-registration could ask some questions of expectant mothers (breast size, shape, growth, etc.) before they check in to determine whether they should be watched for low supply or at least given information about the condition in case they have never heard of it.

Most babies lose some weight after birth, but should be gaining again at the rate of about 1 ounce per day starting on the fifth day of life—and should be back to their birth weight by their 2-week visit to the pediatrician. Weight loss of more than 10% during that first 2 weeks warrants a closer look. Is baby able to transfer milk well from the breast?

An IBCLC who can weigh your baby with a very sensitive scale can help you determine how much milk he is getting during a feeding, but keep in mind that this is only a snapshot of one feeding and should be followed up. While pumping or hand expression does not reliably indicate how much milk a mother is expressing (a soft, sweet-smelling, efficiently feeding baby will usually remove more milk than a hard plastic pump with a motor and a vacuum), if you can express more than a few milliliters of milk after breast-feeding, this could also be a sign that your baby isn't removing milk from your breasts as well as he should. Find a skilled practitioner and check for posterior tongue tie if there is any question that your baby is not removing milk from your breasts effectively. Over time, this understimulation can lead to a significant milk supply deficit because the body is tricked into thinking that less milk is needed.

Weight gain over time, especially during the first month, is an important indicator of how much milk your baby is getting and whether it's adequate for growth and development. As mentioned already, a baby should be back to his birth weight at 2 weeks of age, gaining about an ounce a day starting on day 5. Until 4 months of age, an average gain of 4–7 ounces per week is expected; this gain usually slows down a bit between months 4 and 6 and averages

4–5 ounces a week. For the rest of baby's first year and with the introduction of nutrient-dense, complimentary foods, a breastfed baby should average 2–4 ounces of growth each week (Riordan & Wambach, 2010).

It is common for new parents to want to see their baby "scoring high" on the growth chart curves. We all want our babies to be "the best," right? However, it is important to remember that a baby growing on the 5th percentile curve of a growth chart is *still growing* if he follows that curve. He's just a smaller baby than most other babies his age. There is no need to push him to weigh more than everyone else. Being on the 50th or 95th percentile curves only mean that these babies weigh more than half or 95% of other babies at the same age. A healthy baby can spend his whole infancy at the bottom of the growth chart, so long as he's maintaining adequate growth and development. Ask yourself: are you at the top of the percentile charts for height and weight? Do you want to be?

An outstanding resource that offers a growth calculator and comprehensive, evidence-based information about how much milk your baby should be taking each day can be found at *http://kellymom.com/bf/pumpingmoms/pumping/milkcalc/.* I especially like that this resource cautions against gauging a baby's needs by how vigorously he goes for a bottle.

Even a satisfied baby may "chow down" if a bottle is offered because, even when he is nutritionally full, a baby may still have sucking needs to meet. This is so easy to do at his mother's breast because nutritive (taking in food) and non-nutritive (comfort) suckling regulate a baby's intake there. A bottle teat is designed to deliver its contents quickly in response to the slightest vacuum, so there is little opportunity for a baby to signal he's done eating if he still wants to suck for comfort. Simply stated, a baby who vigorously accepts a bottle may do so for reasons other than hunger.

In addition, understand that a baby being fed a breastmilk substitute will cue to feed less frequently than one who is being fed breastmilk only. This is not a reflection on the adequacy of the breastmilk but on the inability of the baby's body to easily use the substitute—it takes longer to digest. A breastfed baby (or breastmilk fed—fed human milk other than directly from the breast) should be taking about 2–3 ounces 8–12 times a day after his tenth day of life. Some babies take less more frequently, and this is okay, too.

When Breastfeeding Is Not Enough

When it becomes obvious that your baby is not thriving on breast-feeding alone, you and your pediatrician may determine that you need to offer supplemental feedings so your baby receives enough calories and nutrition to grow and develop appropriately. Your first choice, of course, is your expressed milk if it is available. Even some mothers with IGT find that they are able to express some milk in addition to what their babies are getting at the breast. This additional stimulation can also be good for your milk supply. Perhaps you are skilled at hand-expressing and find that you are able to get more milk from your breasts than a pump is able to give you. See the Resource Chapter at the end of this book for a terrific instructional video on hand expression.

> *For the first few days after birth, your baby receives colostrum, a thick, concentrated milk from your breasts. Because colostrum is made during pregnancy, when the hormone setting in your body is different than it is postpartum, and because colostrum only needs to be available in very small amounts in order for a baby to get enough, there is no evidence that even a mother with IGT or one who will not ultimately make enough milk for her baby should have to supplement in the first 48–72 hours after birth. The colostrum should be enough. However, if the baby cannot adequately transfer this colostrum (because of problems with his own oral anatomy), immediate supplementation may be necessary, but this is not because you don't have the capacity to make enough milk; it is because your baby is having trouble removing what you are producing. The need to supplement within the first 48–72 hours after birth does not confirm a milk supply issue in the mother. Also, failure to provide the breasts with adequate and frequent stimulation during that window of time (such as when the baby is supplemented and, therefore, not willing to latch on and suckle) can further compromise a suboptimal milk-making situation.*

If you are more comfortable using a pump to express your milk, first make sure the pump you've chosen is one that will actually do the job you need it to do; not all pumps are created equally. Be particularly wary of pumps that are provided via insurance coverage in the United States. IBCLCs and mothers are finding that these pumps meet only minimum standards for effectiveness and performance. They are less likely to be suitable for the unique needs of a mother with IGT.

Single-User or Multi-User?

It is important to note that the Food and Drug Administration, which oversees the safety and effectiveness of breast pumps in the United States, does not recognize the phrase "hospital grade," which historically has been used (and is often still used) to describe large, durable, multiuser breast pumps. Instead, look for the labels *single-user* or *multi-user*. A single-user breast pump is exactly that; it is designed for use by one person, just like other personal products, such as a toothbrush or a swimsuit. While it may be tempting to save some money by borrowing or purchasing a single-user breast pump from another mother, even a mother whose milk you might consider feeding to your baby, this is strongly discouraged for safety reasons unless the pump was manufactured to be used by more than one user (usually with a new kit of flanges, tubes, and collection containers for each user).

How Strong and How Fast?

The effectiveness of a breast pump is related to how strong a vacuum it can create and how many times it cycles (through suction and release) in a minute. Obviously, the pumps that most closely approximate the suction and pacing of an efficiently feeding baby will do the best job of removing the milk in your breasts. Because an infant feeds with suction levels between 50 and 220 mm Hg (millimeters of mercury, the common measure of negative pressure that is created by a baby's suckling or the vacuum of the pump), choosing a pump that is able to duplicate this rate is best (Slusser & Frantz, 2001). Suction levels lower than 150 mm Hg may not be effective at removing milk from the breast, and suction rates over 220 mm Hg may cause pain (Roche-Paull, 2012).

After you choose a pump that is capable of this level of suction (most likely a high-quality, double-electric pump), experiment with the suction strength to see how you get the most milk out. Not all mothers will get the most milk at the highest level of suction. If you're unsure about how well your pump sucks (pun intended!), an IBCLC may be able to help you by testing it with a pressure gauge.

The number of times the pump cycles in a minute is another consideration in the choice of an effective breast pump. Because a baby suckles 74 times in 1 minute on average, with a range between 40 and 126 cycles each minute (Zoppou, Barry, & Mercer, 1997), a pump that can approximate this pace range may work best.

Again, after you ensure that your pump is capable of cycling fast enough (high-quality, double-electric pumps are most likely to be able to do this), experiment with your pump to see if you are most comfortable with a slower or faster cycling rate.

You may find that you can get more milk out at less than the fastest cycle speed. To measure the cycling frequency of your pump, set a timer for 60 seconds (1 minute) and count the number of clicks (one cycle of suction and release is equal to one click) that you hear from the pump in that time.

Making Pumping More Comfortable with IGT

Breasts that have IGT may be large or small, with dense, milk-making tissue unevenly distributed throughout the breast or located only in the area directly behind the nipple/areola, which is often the cause of breasts that have a tubular shape.

With tubular-shaped breasts, any glandular tissue may be forced into the pump flange (the trumpet-shaped piece of your pump) during pumping. While this ensures that the glandular tissue will be stimulated well, it may also be a source of extreme discomfort if the pump flange does not fit properly. If lubrication of the pump flange with coconut or olive oil doesn't relieve persistent discomfort, the pump flange may be the wrong size. Many mothers with IGT have found that they need a larger sized pump flange than the one that comes standard with most breast pumps. Some have also discovered that a soft, flexible flange with a little "give" allows that herniated glandular tissue to be adequately stimulated without causing pain.

For mothers with "spotty" glandular tissue that may be located in seemingly random spots around the breasts, effective pumping may require a "hands-on" approach. Many mothers with IGT can identify with accuracy where their milk-making tissue is in their breasts—it's in the spots that feel different between feeds or that feel more solid and dense when you feel and squeeze your breasts.

When feeding your baby or pumping your breasts, you will want to make sure that you are adequately stimulating these areas of glandular tissue. One strategy is to think of a straight line that runs from the spot of glandular tissue directly out to the pump flange. For example, if you feel a dense spot in the lower, outside part of your breast, you might try aiming the back of your pump flange at your opposite elbow, just as if when you're feeding your baby, you might try latching him on with his chin pointed toward the area of your breast that has milk. This may help to more effectively drain those areas of your breasts and encourage them to keep making as much milk as they can.

While pumping, you might also consider breast massage. Jones, Dimmock, and Spencer (2001) found that mothers of preterm babies who were pumping milk for them were able to express more milk when they also employed breast massage during pumping. A hands-free pumping bra may make this technique easier as the study also found that pumping both breasts at the same time resulted in a higher milk output than pumping each breast individually in sequence.

Be sure to experiment with breast massage techniques that work best for your unique anatomy. You may find that massaging the areas where you feel breast tissue maximizes your output or that handling your entire breast while pumping helps you yield more milk. Whatever works is the best technique for you!

> *I wish every mother newly diagnosed with IGT could know that she CAN breastfeed, that using supplement does not make her less of a nursing mother, and that while less than ideal, using supplementers at the breast can still create a very satisfying emotional experience for mother and baby.*

When You Need More Milk than You're Able to Make

Although some women with IGT may be able to coax the tissue they do have to make enough milk to exclusively feed their babies by combining feedings at the breast with additional pumping or

hand-expressing, many cannot. The decision about what to supplement your milk with may be an easy one for you, or it may require
some deeper consideration.

Commercially Prepared Breastmilk Substitutes

Before the introduction of animal-milk-based alternatives to
breastmilk for babies who could not receive their mother's milk
(for whatever reason), wet-nursing was the norm and, without
dispute, the safest method of feeding these babies.

The development and improvement of refrigeration and sanitation
practices, as well as increased knowledge about the composition
of animal milks and human milk led to the creation of breastmilk
substitutes for feeding human babies. These served as an additional
option for families whose babies did not receive their mother's milk
(for whatever reason).

In the late 1800s, early versions of these milks contained cow's
milk, wheat flour, malt flour, and potassium bicarbonate. Later, oils,
minerals (such as iron), vitamins, and fatty acids were added. The
ratio of milk proteins (casein and whey) was also adjusted in an
attempt to approximate the ratio found in human milk. Breastmilk
substitutes with a soy protein base were concocted during the
mid-1900s to provide an option for families whose babies could
not tolerate the cow's dairy-based mixtures (U.S. Department of
Agriculture [USDA], 2004).

Choosing a breastmilk substitute may seem like a complicated
process because of the myriad marketing claims that are made

by manufacturers to convince you that one product is superior or better suited for your baby or situation than another (see Chapter 6 for more information about these marketing practices).

However, it is important to recognize that, for the most part, all of these products are created equal—they have to be in order to meet the requirements of the *Codex Alimentarius* Commission, which are explained in the following section. Claims such as "more like breastmilk" or "gentler to baby's tummy" are false, misleading, and not based in scientific evidence.

One category of breastmilk substitutes that isn't created equal are the organic options. Many families will feel better offering an organic option if a commercially prepared breastmilk substitute is necessary.

An excellent resource for help in understanding each ingredient and choosing the best alternative for your baby can be found at this link: *http://foodbabe.com/2013/05/28/how-to-find-the-safest-organic-infant-formula/#more-13333.*

If you are unsure about which commercially prepared breastmilk substitute is best for your baby, seek guidance from your pediatrician.

Low Milk Supply? You have options!

Find what works for you!

You do not have to give up breastfeeding if you have low supply.

There are many things you can do to maximize your supply, and many different ways to supplement.

Formula and bottles are options, but they are not the only ones.

Welcoming, supplementing at the breast with a supplemental nursing system such as a Medela SNS or a Lact-Aid supplementer, your own with a feeding tube, cup feeding, haberman special needs feeders, pumping, donor milk, formula.... any combination of these in whatever way works for you.

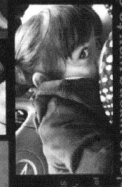

Find an IBCLC, contact your local La Leche League, find an online support group and get the help you need. Every drop of breast milk you can give your baby is beneficial, whether it's 5 ml or 5 oz. a day. You can do this.

Breastfeeding does not have to be ALL OR NOTHING.

http://kellymom.com
http://www.mobimotherhood.org
http://www.bmi/bm/
http://www.drjacknewman.com/
http://www.http://lowmilk-supply.org/

There's no *wrong* way to do it.
The most important thing is that *the baby gets fed!*

Figure 10. Graphic courtesy Jessica Butanda and Nyssa Retter. Used with permission.

Homemade Breastmilk Substitutes

Many of us have family members who remember (or even still recommend!) homemade mixtures of evaporated milk, corn syrup, and vitamin drops; perhaps we or our parents were fed these recipes alongside some breastfeeding. Worldwide, organizations that seek to protect the health of infants recommend against the use of homemade mixtures.

Milks from other animals, such as goats, may put babies at risk for kidney problems or other serious medical issues, especially within the first month of life. "Milks" made from nuts, plants, or grains, even when fortified, may be deficient in the energy (calories), fat, protein, or other nutrients that are necessary for growth and development.

Regardless of the strong guidance against their use, the Internet offers countless recipes for homemade breastmilk substitutes for those who seek to avoid the available commercially prepared ones and choose not to use donor human milk.

If you choose to take this approach to supplementing your baby, be sure to review the standards set forth by the *Codex Alimentarius* Commission, which was established by the United Nations in the 1960s to regulate food safety and consumer protection on an international level. These standards include, but are not limited to the following:

◆ Breastmilk substitutes must be made from cow's milk or other animal milks that have been proven suitable for infant feeding. All ingredients must be gluten-free.

- Breastmilk substitutes must meet requirements for energy provided per 100 mL (enough but not too many calories).

- Breastmilk substitutes must meet requirements for protein, fats, and carbohydrates in specified amounts (enough but not too much)

- Breastmilk substitutes must meet requirements for specific vitamins, minerals, and fatty acids (enough but not too much).

- Breastmilk substitutes may include other ingredients that have been scientifically demonstrated to be suitable for infant feeding in sufficient amounts to affect specific outcomes or to provide substances found in breastmilk.

- Breastmilk substitutes must comply with purity and hygiene specifications in the manufacturing process.

- Breastmilk substitutes must be monitored for any additives or contaminants, such that fillers or pesticide residues do not exceed maximum allowable levels.

The full text of the *Codex Alimentarius* Commission's recommendations can be found at this link: *http://www.codexalimentarius.org/input/download/standards/.../CXS_072e.pdf.*

Special Situations
If your baby is intolerant of cow's milk-based breastmilk substitutes, you may consider using soy protein-based products; however, these may not be the best option in all cases.

Work closely with your pediatrician to determine whether a soy-based breastmilk substitute is the superior alternative for your baby. Some questions and answers about these products can be found at this link: _http://www.askdrsears.com/topics/feeding-infants-toddlers/bottle-feeding/soy-formulas._

Some babies may show signs of allergy or intolerance when fed anything but breastmilk. These symptoms may include eczema, rashes (including but not limited to the diaper area), gas, pasty or thick "peanut butter" stools that may be difficult for the baby to pass, stools with blood or mucus in them, fussiness or colic, congestion, wheezing, or ear infections.

In a baby who is being fed both mother's milk (and/or the breast-milk of another mother) and cow's milk-based or soy breastmilk substitutes, it may be difficult to determine whether the baby is reacting to the breastmilk substitutes or if he is a generally reactive baby who might be having trouble with something in your (or your milk donor's) diet.

One way to try to sort this out is to save the milk you are able to express for a few days until you have enough to supplement your baby's feedings at your breasts for at least one full day. Feed your baby only your milk, then watch closely. While one full day may not be long enough to conclusively determine whether your baby is struggling with his supplement to your milk, many families are able to note a significant enough difference in their babies after a 24-hour trial (if you're producing enough milk to accomplish a longer trial fairly easily without significantly increasing the amount of supplemental breastmilk substitute you're offering, by all means, do it).

Another option, if it takes you several days to express enough extra milk to account for a whole day or two of supplemental needs, is to use another mother's breastmilk. Information about using donor human milk follows in this chapter.

If, after this breastmilk-only trial, it appears that what you've chosen to supplement with is causing symptoms for your baby, first, try not to berate yourself. It can be easy to fall into a cycle of self-blaming every time your sweet baby is uncomfortable after consuming something other than his favorite meal—your milk!

Remember that your most important priority is to *feed your baby*, and you're doing the best your body will let you to give him your milk. Second, do your research and consider the alternatives that are available to you. There are hypoallergenic manufactured breast-milk substitutes; these are separately regulated by government agencies and are included, with products for premature babies and those with rare metabolic disorders, in a category called "exempt infant formulas." Because of their cost, these products are intended for use only when the medical indication to do so is clear.

There are two types of breastmilk substitutes that are considered hypoallergenic: hydrolysate products, which contain cow's milk proteins that are broken down, making them less difficult to digest by some babies, and amino-acid-based, or elemental, products; the elemental breastmilk substitutes are milk-free and are made from the building blocks of proteins. If you think your baby needs a hypoallergenic food, talk to your pediatrician about your concerns, and decide together what is best for your baby.

Donor Breastmilk

Under most circumstances in a developed nation (where access to clean water and good hygiene are available), commercially manufactured breastmilk substitutes are considered adequate for providing the nutrients a growing infant requires. However, an increasing number of families are choosing to obtain donor breastmilk to use for supplementation.

There are several reasons a mother might choose to maximize her baby's intake of human milk. These include the following:

- Breastmilk is species-specific; it requires no alteration or manufacturing to be suitable for a human infant.

- Human milk is alive and contains immune properties and other factors that are not added to breastmilk substitutes; this possibly protects infants against certain infectious and non-infectious diseases.

- There is an increased risk of respiratory and gastrointestinal infections for babies not fed breastmilk.

- There is an increased risk of hospitalization for illness for babies not fed breastmilk.

In addition to these physiological reasons for wanting to use donor milk, mothers may have more personal reasons that run deeper than simply ensuring that their baby is fed. In our 2013 study of mothers with lactation difficulties, Penny Liberatos and I were touched by the responses we received to questions about how mothers dealt, emotionally, with their inability to exclusively breastfeed.

Knowing my baby was on donor milk helped me cope because my worst fear was putting her on formula, so donor milk helped me see it as "exclusively" breastfeeding my baby, just not all with my milk.

Getting some donor milk for my first child was very healing.

Deciding to use donor milk the second time around, at eight weeks, was a profound experience. My baby is 20 months now and she is still getting donor milk. Breastfed for 20 months—no small task.

Although I wish that I could exclusively breastfeed, I have learned that I can still nurture my baby at the breast, and that she can still get some breastmilk. I wish milk sharing were more common. I tried really hard to find a donor for my daughter, but didn't really know where to look, and there didn't seem to be anyone in my area that was willing to donate.

I LOVE donor milk and have found lots of support even from "overproducing" moms. It is awesome and I wish I had found it sooner.

Our study also found that, among women who believed they might have IGT, just over a quarter of them used at least some donor milk, which they acquired through milk sharing arrangements with another mother (not from a milk bank—less than 3% of respondents reported using banked milk as a supplement).

Donor milk that has come from a milk bank, such as those operated by the Human Milk Banking Association of North America (find more information at this link: _https://www.hmbana.org/_), has been collected according to specific standards, screened, pooled with the milk of other donors, pasteurized, and tested/cultured before being distributed by prescription. Banked milk is a potentially lifesaving option for unwell or premature babies whose mothers are unable to provide enough breastmilk for them because breastmilk substitutes dramatically increase the risk of a serious gastrointestinal condition called necrotizing enterocolitis (NEC). However, for healthy babies, long-term use of banked milk may not be practical; it requires a prescription, and it can be very expensive, perhaps $3–$5 per ounce.

For the families that would prefer to use donor breastmilk as a supplement, mother-to-mother milk sharing is an option that is increasing in popularity. The advent of Internet-facilitated milk sharing is to credit for this increase, but also raises concerns for health agencies and families. Akre, Gribble, and Minchin (2011) addressed these concerns in their article, "Milk Sharing: From Private Practice to Public Pursuit" _(http://www.ncbi.nlm.nih.gov/pmc/articles/PMC3151205/)._ Gribble and Hausman (2012), in their article "Milk Sharing and Formula Feeding: Infant Feeding Risks in Comparative Perspective?" _(http://www.ncbi.nlm.nih.gov/pmc/articles/PMC3395287/)._ simplified and discussed how to minimize the inherent risks of any method of feeding one's baby.

A family that is considering using donor milk from another mother should consider these research articles required reading for the decision-making process. The risks that are discussed include:

- Contamination with pathogens

◆ Contamination with chemicals

◆ Poor hygiene and improper storage

◆ Health risks associated with use of formula

◆ Likelihood of transmission of HIV via donated milk

The largest Internet milk-sharing network, Human Milk 4 Human Babies *(http://hm4hb.net/faq/),* offers comprehensive, specific guidelines for minimizing any risks associated with mother-to-mother milk sharing, including talking points and questions to ask your potential donors, medical tests you might wish to order for your potential donors, and an at-home method of pasteurizing the milk you receive if you wish to. The Resource Chapter in this book offers additional places to find more information.

> *I used donor milk from my best friend and supplemented at the breast. At almost 3 years old, my daughter still nurses several times a day and at night. I finally got the extended nursing relationship that I have desperately wanted, and thanks to donor milk, I didn't have to feel guilty about supplementing and giving my baby less than the best.*

I Can't Get Past the "Ick Factor" of Feeding My Baby Someone Else's Milk

A recent study was released with great fanfare. It revealed that breastmilk *purchased* via the Internet had high levels of bacteria when it was delivered to the recipient (Keim et al., 2013). What most of the media blitz around this article failed to address was that the conditions under which the study was conducted did not remotely approximate "real-life" milk-sharing practices in that milk was *purchased*, not donated. Donors who asked questions about the recipient babies and sought a relationship with the recipient family were disqualified, and milk samples were shipped, not picked up or dropped off, as is common in actual milk-sharing relationships. Shipment often took days, and little or no care was taken to maintain a food-safe temperature of the milk. What was remarkable about this publication, however, was the public's reaction to it. We are currently in a culture that, by and large, finds the sharing of human milk unsanitary and unsafe, even though this is not what the science of *actual* milk sharing between two mothers might reveal.

Our cultural opinion that breastmilk is a bodily fluid rather than a food may contribute to perceptions about milk sharing that are difficult to get over—if not for ourselves then perhaps for those who love us and our babies. Only you can decide which method of supplementation is going to feel the best for you. *If you feel better about using a commercially available breastmilk substitute or something you make yourself, that's okay—just feed your baby.* The availability, non-availability, or attractiveness of donor milk to you does not change the fact that your baby needs to be fed in whatever way is sustainable for you. Before completely dismissing milk sharing as an option, however, ask yourself (or those who oppose your desire to offer another mother's milk to your baby) and your potential milk donors a few questions:

- Is the donor mother feeding her milk to her baby?

- Do you feel better about milk from a woman you've met or

breastmilk substitutes made from the milk of several cows you've never seen? (It's totally okay if you feel better about the cows—some mothers do.)

- How much of your grief and anxiety over having IGT is about the need to feed your baby something other than your own milk? If the answer to this question is "a lot," you may wish to consider reviewing the aforementioned publications with people whose support you desire and having a calm, rational discussion about the risks and benefits of what you choose to feed as a supplement. Being able to feed your baby *what feels best to you* will be a significant step in your healing, and weighing *your own personal value* of the risks and benefits of each alternative will allow you to do that.

Remember as well that no choice you make is all or nothing; you may opt to (or find you have to) supplement partially with donor milk and partially with breastmilk substitutes. Also, if you make one decision and it doesn't sit well with you, you can always change what you're feeding your baby.

For World Milksharing Week in 2012, I participated in a blog carnival of personal stories from families that participated in mother-to-mother milk sharing. My contribution, as well as a link to the other posts in the blog carnival, can be found here: *http://dianaibclc. com/2012/09/24/milksharing-a-story-of-peace-and-healing/.*

Solids as Supplements

Most medical and child health organizations, including the American Academy of Pediatrics (2012), recommend exclusive breastfeeding for about 6 months. Dr. Jack Newman, a Canadian physician and IBCLC, suggests that an earlier introduction of solid foods may be preferable to feeding a breastmilk substitute via bottle for mothers who are producing most of the nutrition that their babies need (Newman & Kernerman, 2009). Keep in mind that, regardless of when the solid foods are offered, they are intended to supplement, not replace, the breastmilk that is also being fed.

In the case of the early introduction of solids, the intent is to offer nutrient-dense food rather than a breastmilk substitute *only* when the majority of the baby's diet is breastmilk (this alternative *would not be appropriate* for the mother who is supplementing with more than a few ounces each day).

While commercially available breastmilk substitutes typically provide 20 calories per ounce, 1 ounce of mashed, ripe avocado provides 50 calories; banana and sweet potato each have 25 calories per ounce, and all are wonderful first foods for your baby. Keep in mind that you want to choose foods that will promote growth, not simply create a feeling of fullness in your baby. Also, remember that a baby who is consuming solid food may also need some water to drink. If you think that the early introduction of solid foods might be an appropriate option for you and your baby, talk to your pediatrician about your concerns, how best to accomplish this, and signs that your baby may be ready to get some of his nutritional needs met with high-calorie solid foods in lieu of a breastmilk substitute.

No matter how you end up piecing together a complete nutritional picture for your baby, pat yourself on the back for a job well done. Whether you can provide 20 ounces of your milk each day or that amount each week doesn't matter quite as much as finding and implementing your best solution to the nutritional problem of low milk supply.

Weigh the pros and cons of all of your options, and feel free to change your course if what you thought would work ends up not being compatible with your baby's needs or your lifestyle. What works for you is your right answer.

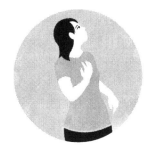

Chapter 6

Breastfeeding Advocacy:
Truth (or Tactics?) That
Can Hurt

B reastfeeding has been identified as a public health concern both nationally and globally. Organizations such as the World Health Organization (WHO, 2003) and the American Academy of Pediatrics (AAP, 2012) have offered policy statements that uphold breastfeeding as the normal and optimal method of infant and young child feeding.

In the United States, the Department of Health and Human Services and Centers for Disease Control and Prevention have specified target rates for breastfeeding initiation, exclusivity, and duration in its Healthy People goals for 2020. While 76.9% of new mothers in the United States initiate breastfeeding, only 43.5% are breastfeeding at all at 6 months. These mothers may be mixed-feeding with breastmilk substitutes or offering solids. At 12 months, only 25.5% of mothers are breastfeeding at all (Centers for Disease Control and Prevention [CDC], 2012). These figures are well under the Healthy People 2020 targets of 81.9% of babies initiating breast-feeding, 60.6% of babies still breastfeeding at 6 months, and 34.1% of babies breastfeeding at all at 12 months of age (HHS, Healthy People 2020, 2012).

In an effort to increase breastfeeding rates, countless organiza-tions and individuals have created and disseminated messages that may be characterized as breastfeeding advocacy, promotion, or support. However, for the mother who cannot produce a full milk supply for her baby, these messages are more likely received like a kick in the stomach—an attack that adds insult to the injury already experienced by her inability to breastfeed exclusively despite her intent and desire to do so.

I wish full supply moms would stop blaming and shaming low supply moms for needing to supplement.

Exclusive breastfeeding is physiologically impossible for many women with IGT, no matter how hard they try or how committed to breastfeeding they might be. This dichotomy between wanting what she has been taught is best for her baby and what she's able to provide may be a very difficult one for a mother with IGT to accept. Messages from well-meaning health care providers—perhaps the same ones that told you throughout your pregnancy that you should consider exclusive breastfeeding—that not breastfeeding "isn't the end of the world" or "isn't a big deal" may feel like patronizing lies.

Even worse, the advocacy messages of various breastfeeding promotion campaigns (organized or random) that permeate the "mommy blogosphere" and social media platforms might feel like personal attacks on you. You *wanted* to breastfeed, to give your precious baby the very best of everything, and those messages, which practically criminalize artificial infant feeding, are of no help to you. They might even contribute to the growing sense of anger, guilt, or shame that you're already experiencing.

Being unable to sustain my child, and feeling that my body was broken was devastating for me. No one had ever told me that a failure to produce milk was even possible unless someone "gave up." I was judged, guilted and made to feel like I was ignorant and lazy by friends, family and medical professionals and it was not until I found the information buried deep beneath the sea of "all women can breastfeed as long as they try hard enough" that I began to heal.

Advocacy?

It's clear that a baby fed at his mother's breast will be less likely to suffer the same health risks that befall babies who are not breastfed.[3] Some, but perhaps not all, of these health risks are also avoided when a baby is *breastmilk fed,* which is the term used to describe how mothers who exclusively pump (EP-ers) or those who supplement their own milk supply with human donor milk feed their babies.

Mothers who combine feeding at the breast with feedings given in some other way (perhaps because of a return to work or school, or in cases of adoptive breastfeeding or low milk supply) are both breastfeeding and breastmilk feeding. There is growing awareness in breastfeeding research that breastfeeding and breastmilk feeding are not identical. This awareness rightly considers that there is more to breastfeeding than just the milk!

Health outcomes may be affected by *how* a baby is fed, not just by *what* he is being fed. It is both possible and advisable to approximate physiologically normal feeding, even when exclusive breastfeeding is not possible. While campaigns to boost breastfeeding rates are rooted in the intent to emphasize the real differences between breastfeeding/breastmilk feeding and artificial feeding, sometimes the messages of these campaigns are insensitive and not even completely based in evidence. You've seen them—perhaps, before your baby was born, you've even propagated them.

---

3   There are lots of places where you can learn about the risks of not breastfeeding if you haven't already. The resources cited in this chapter are among them. Because this book is about focusing on what we *can* accomplish and not on what we *cannot* do, the risks of not breastfeeding do not appear here.

DID YOU EVER WONDER WHAT'S IN... ?

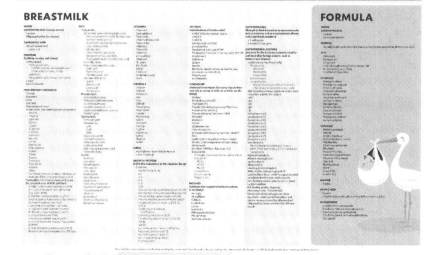

Breastmilk has more of
the good things babies need

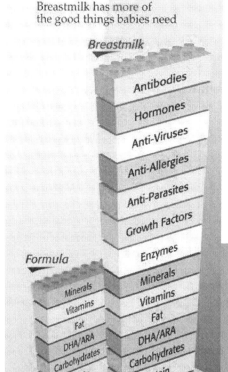

Figure 11. A comparison of the components of species-specific human milk with a plant- or animal-protein-based breastmilk substitute can remind us of how precious every drop of milk we're able to provide truly is.

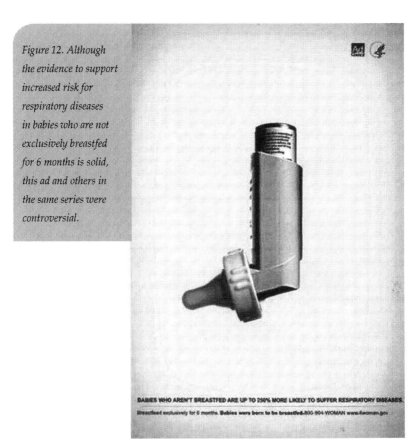

Figure 12. Although the evidence to support increased risk for respiratory diseases in babies who are not exclusively breastfed for 6 months is solid, this ad and others in the same series were controversial.

What's the best milk after Julie's?

Julie breastfed her daughter because she knew it was the normal milk for her baby, and she had great support. When she finished, she didn't need to use a breastmilk substitute at all. Julie chose breastfeeding as she knows it has been around for thousands of years. For Julie and her baby the best choice was continued breastfeeding.

According to the World Health Organisation (WHO)

2nd choice is mother's own milk given via cup or bottle
3rd is breastmilk from a milk bank or wet nurse
4th and last is Infant formula

To find out if human milk is the best milk for you, visit analyticalarmadillo.co.uk

Figure 13. What this meme doesn't clarify is that the fourth option is superior to not feeding your baby at all when the first three options are not available.

Figure 14. While this meme is obviously intended to debunk the myth that making enough milk is difficult and to encourage mothers to trust their bodies (correct guidance for most mothers), it feeds the once-popular "if she can gestate, she can lactate" line of thinking that we now know isn't necessarily true.

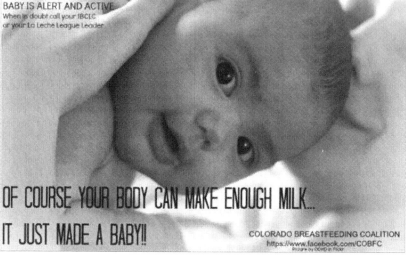

Figure 15. This one misses the mark: skilled lactation help can identify breastfeeding problems, but the solutions to those problems will differ from mother to mother (and may include feeding the baby something other than breastmilk). Let's consider whether this meme would have a similarly inflammatory effect if, instead of formula, it pointed a finger at supplementation? Who could argue that, in some cases, supplementation is a solution to a breastfeeding problem?

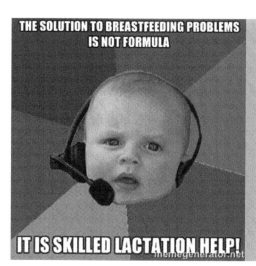

Making Milk

is Easy!

10 Steps to make plenty of milk

1 Frequent feeds, not formula.
The more often you feed, the more milk you make. If you give formula, your body will make less milk.

2 All you need is breastmilk!
The American Academy of Pediatrics recommends that your baby have a diet of purely breastmilk for the first 6 months—no other food or drink is needed.

3 Feed early and often.
Feed at the earliest signs of hunger: if baby's awake, sucking on hands, moving his mouth or eyes, or stretching.

4 If he didn't swallow, he didn't eat.
Looking and listening for signs of swallowing will help you know that your baby's getting enough.

5 Say 'No' to pacifiers and bottles,
at least in the first 4 weeks. Pacifiers may hide the signs of hunger. The American Academy of Pediatrics recommends that you should not use a pacifier for the first month if you are breastfeeding. If your baby has problems sucking, check with a lactation specialist about how to feed him without using a bottle.

6 Sleep near your baby and nurse lying down.
You can rest while you feed your baby!

7 Have baby's mouth open wide like a shout, with lips flipped out.
Help your baby open his mouth as wide as possible. He should be directly facing you: "belly to belly, chest to chest, and his chin should touch the breast." Proper positioning keeps you both comfortable. If you're having trouble with latch, get help promptly.

8 Watch the baby, not the clock.
Feed your baby when she's hungry, and switch sides when swallowing slows down or she takes herself off the breast.

9 Go everywhere!
Plan to take your newborn everywhere with you for the first several weeks.

10 Don't wait to ask for help, if you need it.
If you wait too long to get the help you need, it may be harder to breastfeed. Stick with it – it's worth it!

Massachusetts Breastfeeding Coalition
254 Conant Road
Weston, MA 02493
www.massbreastfeeding.org

© 2011 Massachusetts Breastfeeding Coalition

Figure 16.
Again, for most mothers, the guidance offered here is true and can also help maximize milk output when there is a preglandular or postglandular milk-making problem.

Yet, the message that "making milk is easy" can be devastating for those mothers who worked very hard to make enough milk for their babies.

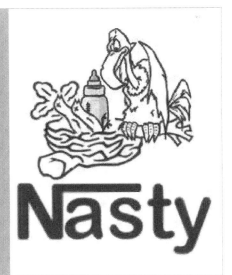

Figure 17. It's important to differentiate between efforts against the predatory marketing practices of breastmilk-substitute manufacturers and the breastmilk substitutes themselves.

Graphics like these don't point fingers at mothers who need to or choose to use a breastmilk substitute. They instead take aim at the companies that seek profits from their sale and market them to mothers who have no feeding issues whatsoever.

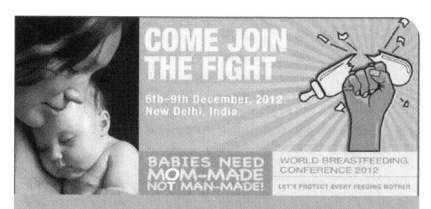

Figure 18. In a developing nation, like India, breastfeeding can mean the difference between life and death for infants born there. The same could be said for babies born in poverty in developed nations. Is this meme attacking mothers in developed nations whose breasts do not function properly? No, but the anti-bottle message can feel accusatory to the mother who has to or chooses to use a "man-made, not mom-made" breastmilk substitute.

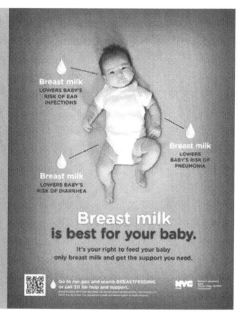

Figure 19. While this graphic may at first discourage mothers who cannot exclusively breastfeed their babies, a deeper reading reveals that "It's your right to feed your baby only breastmilk and get the support you need."

Isn't this a call to action for more research into why lactation doesn't always work? Doesn't society at large have a responsibility to fulfill that right to exclusive breastmilk and support for every mother and baby?

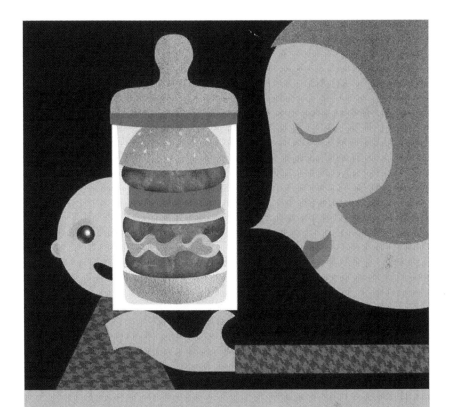

Figure 20. The notion that breastmilk substitutes are "junk food" doesn't really help anyone. This graphic, too, fails to account for the fact that a baby fed with a substitute is going to be healthier than a baby not fed at all! Whether the breastmilk substitute was a mother's choice or the only option she was left with matters less than the fact that her baby is fed a food that will enable him to develop and thrive.

I have learned that breastfeeding is about so much more than milk! I may feel disappointed with my breasts, but my baby seeks comfort from being near to (and latched on) my breasts every day.

"Just One Bottle"

When you see messages that promote breastfeeding by disparaging artificial (formula) feeding, you might feel insulted, attacked, and marginalized. Although it is true that just one bottle can have health repercussions (Walker, n.d.), mothers who struggle with the early, severe milk-production problems that often accompany IGT are acutely aware of the health repercussions that come with *not feeding the baby!*

Let's imagine for a minute that we have a medical condition that requires medication—good health practices, like diet and exercise, don't make this condition go away. Perhaps this medication is controversial because it has side effects for some people, or maybe there are health campaigns against it because people who aren't sick get their doctors to prescribe it. Maybe this medicine seems to make life more convenient, or maybe some people get it for free through their insurance, which is a lot easier than the good health practices that *would* help those people who ought to but don't want to follow them. The sick people who *need* the medication don't feel guilty for using it because they already know they've done (with comprehensive support from their health care providers) everything they can to avoid using it, right?

Why is the use of a breastmilk substitute when full lactation is physiologically impossible (for whatever reason) different? Perhaps these reasons come to mind:

- Awareness that failure to fully meet a baby's needs through breastfeeding is possible is increasing, but not yet universal, so the message "may be you didn't try hard enough" is bound to come from someone. Maybe you even worry that in your exhausted postpartum haze, *you* actually derailed your own breastfeeding experience. You probably didn't.

- There are so many reasons for low milk production. Most of them can be prevented or mitigated with qualified, comprehensive health care and breastfeeding support. Does someone think you didn't get good support? Do you doubt the expertise of the people who were supposed to help you get breastfeeding off to a good start?

- The use of human milk from donor mothers is increasing among families who are unable to produce enough milk. This is great for those who choose to or are able to practice this option, but may be discouraging for families that are not comfortable with it or can't find suitable donors (see Chapter 5 for more information on using donor human milk).

- Because there is no conclusive diagnostic process or criteria for IGT, there may always be doubt that you really couldn't breastfeed, and health messages that promote exclusive breastfeeding may remind you of that doubt.

One strategy you might find helpful is to ask yourself, "who is this message intended for?" Health communicators don't prefer to use scare tactics or shaming techniques to discourage unhealthy behaviors. If a photo of a diseased lung never encouraged someone to quit smoking or pleas from mothers who lost children to drunk driving accidents never gave someone pause before getting behind the wheel after a few drinks, such campaigns wouldn't be used. Keep in mind that every campaign has a target audience: potential consumers of health-promoting behaviors or goods. In the case of infant feeding, expectant and new mothers (and, increasingly, those who influence them, such as the babies' fathers and grandmothers) are the target audience.

If a woman has breasts and gives birth, she's a potential breastfeeder, a potential consumer or practitioner of a proven health-promoting, disease-preventing behavior. Let's dissect part of that last sentence: "if a woman has breasts." Sure, women with IGT have breasts, and often, these breasts look quite lovely—full and large. However, until the baby arrives, there is no confirmation that they are functional or that there aren't factors outside of the breasts, such as hormonal issues, that affect whether or how effectively the milk factory does its job. Are these messages for you? If you decide that they aren't (hint: they're probably not), why do they hurt so much?

> *Some members of the breastfeeding support community struggle with social movements to accept and even encourage the routine feeding of breastmilk substitutes, for the sake of social propriety, to not make the non-breastfeeding mother feel bad. The emphasis in these movements is on not judging families for their choice of infant feeding method, whether there was an intent to breastfeed that got derailed or no desire to breastfeed whatsoever. This assumes that there was indeed, a choice to be made, that the healthy option was also the easy option. Often, the social determinants that surround a family's infant feeding decision don't make breastfeeding the easy option, so presenting infant feeding as a "lifestyle" choice rather than as a public health issue becomes complicated.*

> What this attitude of tolerance also fosters, albeit unintentionally, is a cultural acceptance that breastmilk substitutes are "good enough." If this is the truth, if there is nothing to be gained from improving breastfeeding rates, where is the impetus to understand why some women can't breastfeed? Lactation research is largely underfunded, and this may be the unfortunate reason: there is no health problem if the alternative is "good enough." Indeed, no family should be shamed or judged when the healthy choice isn't the easy choice, but it is possible to be more nuanced in our language: substitutes are a viable alternative when breastfeeding or breastmilk are not possible or desired, but they are not the norm. Our discourse should reflect the truth so that real solutions to the barriers to breastfeeding can be researched and implemented. This is not commentary on the quality of the mother who feeds her baby a breastmilk substitute; it returns the focus to where it belongs: on the societal responsibility to make the healthy choice the easy choice.

Guilt vs. Regret

If anything is true about motherhood, it's that once the baby is born (or even before!), mothers find themselves overcome with the sheer breadth of their new responsibility. Every mother wants her baby to be happy, healthy, and successful, and she will go to lengths she never imagined in order to protect and nurture her child. At the same time, no one—parent or otherwise—wants to feel bad; as humans, we do our best to avoid (so we don't have to cope with) unpleasant feelings. Two especially unpleasant feelings that accompany being human are *guilt* and *regret*. They are similar but not the same; being able to distinguish between the two can go a long way in coping with or healing from situations where things don't go the way we intended for them to go, such as when breastfeeding doesn't work.

Dictionary.com *(http://dictionary.reference.com/)* offers us a starting point for understanding guilt and regret with the definitions of these two words:

> *Guilt: A feeling of responsibility or remorse for some offense, crime, wrong, etc., whether real or imagined*
>
> *Regret: A feeling of sadness, repentance, or disappointment over something that has happened or been done*

Both guilt and regret are feelings. Guilt appears to be a feeling associated with a commission of something wrong or bad: something that the person feeling guilt did (or didn't do). The feeling of regret, which is very similar to guilt (with "repentance" being part of regret) seems to follow a circumstance: something that has happened to the person feeling the emotion.

There's another difference, too. According to a recent study (Wagner, Handke, Dörfel, & Walter, 2012), guilt, but not regret, occurs in social/ interpersonal contexts. Subjects in their study only felt guilt when there was some social dimension involved. How does this apply to our feelings about not being able to exclusively breastfeed? In a nutshell: if you were not surrounded by messages that "breast is best" or that not breastfeeding is akin to a criminal offense—if breastfeeding was a behavior that was done in social isolation—you might feel regret if things didn't go well, but you would be less likely to feel guilt.

Does breastfeeding, or any infant care practice, take place in a vacuum? If you're old enough to remember the film *The Blue Lagoon*, maybe you'll recall that Brooke Shields's character, a young teen on a remote island with her boyfriend, had no idea that she was even pregnant. Instinct took over in the absence of social observations and support, but is that what happens in our culture? Absolutely not! That social dimension is an integral (and good!) part of becoming a mother in our culture, but it makes the differentiation of guilt from regret even muddier.

Did you choose or cause your baby to be denied your breastmilk? Of course not! This is something that, for whatever reason (physiology, inadequate support, lack of information), *happened to you*. Do you (or did you) judge those who choose to not breastfeed? Might a more compassionate attitude toward those mothers, regardless of what you know about their situation, help you soften the judgments you heap upon yourself? Who determines when a mother has "tried hard enough" or whether the support she got was competent and comprehensive enough to truly protect a breastfeeding relationship?

I thought I got "over" my (mainly emotional) challenges of not being able to breastfeed my first child, until I discovered that I am currently pregnant with my second child. Just thinking about breastfeeding gets my heart rate up. One side of my brain tells me: go and get information now. But the other side tells me, "don't even go there, you know the struggles of last time, just formula feed this time and enjoy your baby right from the start." It's a very confusing and overwhelming topic for me…still.

The WHO Code and You

For much of Western culture, breastfeeding is considered an "elective" behavior. A substitute exists that permits babies to thrive in the absence of their mother's own milk, regardless of whether that absence is due to circumstance or personal choice.

Complicating this issue and likely contributing to the "criminalization" of mothers who do not breastfeed is the fact that this substitute doesn't simply *exist*—it is *promoted* for *profit* with *no regulation* in countries that have not voluntarily elected to enforce the criteria set forth by the World Health Organizaion's International Code of Marketing of Breastmilk Substitutes (WHO, 1981), also called the WHO Code. In these countries, infant formula companies recognize that their product competes for market share with breastmilk.

In the absence of legislation that ensures that the marketing and distribution of products that substitute for human milk are scientifically based and honest, formula companies can—and do—run amok with their claims that their formula (or bottles) are "most like mom," "closer to breastmilk," or otherwise protective of health—or even that they are *better than breastmilk.*

The public health initiatives that uphold the WHO Code to protect breastfeeding (and thus, the health of babies and their mothers) must work against these marketing messages of formula companies. Mothers for whom breastfeeding didn't work as planned or who make the informed choice to not breastfeed are caught in the crossfire.

About the WHO Code

The World Health Organization's Code of Marketing of Breastmilk Substitutes (WHO, 1981), also called "The WHO Code," was created to regulate the marketing and distribution of substances and items that substitute for breastfeeding and breastmilk. In countries where the WHO Code is embraced and enforced in the marketing and distribution of breastmilk substitutes (such as artificial baby milks, also called "formula," the bottles/teats that are used to feed these milks, and other products related to infant feeding), the following criteria prevail:

* *Products within the scope of the Code are not be marketed/advertised directly to mothers or the general public.*

* *No samples of products within the scope of the Code are distributed, either directly or indirectly, to pregnant women, mothers, or their family members.*

* *In-store advertising/displays, special discounts/coupons, and free gifts (premiums) of products within the scope of the Code are not permitted.*

In addition, all information that is distributed to health workers by manufacturers of products within the scope of the Code is scientifically based and provides instruction in the safe use of the products. Unless you live in a developing nation, you are surrounded by an entire world of WHO Code violations. What does this mean for the family that sees baby milks, and bottles, teats, and other feeding-related items as necessary? Most importantly, the WHO Code seeks to regulate the marketing and distribution of these items, not the use. Companies are not in violation of the Code by making these products available. Neither is the consumer who purchases them. When Code activists and their messages expose and seek to correct the unethical, predatory marketing practices of certain companies, they're not trying to attack or shame you or your need/choice to use these products.

You might feel like the free containers of breastmilk substitutes and money-saving coupons are good things, and the notion that they should be eliminated is just another way to criminalize the experience you're having. Here's the rub, though: all of those unregulated samples and marketing techniques affect the perceptions of mothers without physiological milk-making problems about their ability to successfully and exclusively breastfeed (Parry, Taylor, Hall-Dardess, Walker, & Labbok, 2013). They also create a lot of confusion when you're trying to figure out how best to feed your baby.

"Most like mom."

"Closer to breastmilk."

"Supplemental formula for breastfed babies."

"Best for babies who switch between bottle and breast."

"Gentle for sensitive babies."

If those statements were accurate and based in scientific evidence, two things would be true. First, hooray! We'd have really clear delineation of which products we should use—the ones that are "the best"! Second, wouldn't there be a movement to ensure that all babies who aren't being exclusively breastfed had access to these "superior" products, not just the ones born to families that can afford them? Consider the Special Supplemental Nutrition Program for Women, Infants, and Children (WIC) in the United States; the breastmilk-substitute brand that is distributed through this government program is determined by each individual state. Exclusive distribution of a given brand in a particular state is awarded to the manufacturer who offers the most competitive bid for that privilege (USDA, 2013).

There is absolutely no evaluation or comparison of the healthfulness or "effectiveness" of any brand, ingredient, or supposed feature when states determine which brand of breastmilk substitute to offer through its WIC program. Let this be a strong message that no formula (bottle, teat, etc.) is inherently superior to another, regardless of what their advertising tells you.

See Chapters 5 and 7 for more information about supplementation.

"But Formula Saved My Baby's Life!"

When we encounter these breastfeeding advocacy (or anti-breastmilk substitute) messages on social media platforms, like Facebook or blogs, we want to stand up for ourselves and educate the individuals or organizations that are spreading those messages.

"My baby could have starved to death had it not been for formula," many mothers share after watching their babies, unable to transfer milk via breastfeeding (because the milk simply wasn't there or for some other reason, such as tongue tie), lose weight, fail to thrive, and in extreme cases, become dehydrated or sick. The bottom line here should be crystal clear.

But, in case it is not, I will spell it out:

> *No person or organization that is interested in health outcomes thinks you should have starved your baby rather than feed him a breastmilk substitute.*

No matter how strong these messages seem to be, no matter how much you think they are directed at you, they are not. Are some of them insensitive or inappropriate? Yes. Does the truth within them, that your breastmilk is, exclusively, the normal first food for your baby, mean that you are somehow a failure because you were unable to provide it? No. How can you convince yourself of that when the messages seem to be everywhere? Focus on what you *can* do, what you *have* done, and what you *are* doing. Can you produce some milk for your baby? Whether a mother makes a full supply of milk or not, some breastmilk is always better than no breastmilk in terms of health outcomes.

Consider replacing the word "formula" with the word "supplementation." *Supplementation* was or is necessary for your baby. *Supplementation* enabled your baby to thrive and develop. No one can argue that, regardless of what you've chosen to supplement with or why you made that choice.

Research is mounting that breastfeeding's goodness isn't just about the milk. Do you feed your baby in a manner that mimics the biological norm of breastfeeding? See the Resource Chapter for more information about how to bottle-feed in a manner that more closely approximates breastfeeding.

Remember that breastfeeding is one (a significant one but still only one) behavior that you can practice to give your baby his best start. Healthy foods when it's time to introduce solids, physical activity, good hygiene, and loving, compassionate care with the physical and emotional attention that your baby/child needs can be offered regardless of what or how your infant was fed.

Even mothers with full milk supplies have challenges. It's so common to find yourself thinking, "this wouldn't happen if I had enough milk to exclusively breastfeed," about everything from an ear infection, a fussy baby, or a diaper rash! Keep in mind that your fellow mothers have plenty else to blame their challenges on:

- *… if I didn't have to go back to work*
- *… if I was raising him in a two-parent home*
- *… if he wasn't born with special needs*
- *… if we had more money/a better house/a better doctor*
- *… if he was a better sleeper*
- *… if I didn't have my own health challenge*
- *… if I had family nearby to help me*
- *… if my family wasn't always at my house*

Knowing that you have done the "very best" that you and your body can do for your baby, whether or not that's the very best that some other mother and her body could do for hers, is a vital step in guarding yourself against messages that might be perceived as hurtful or attacking you. Remember that, even among mothers with full milk supplies, every family is different, and *only you* can decide when you've "tried hard enough" or "done everything" to make breastfeeding or lactating work. Taking honest stock of *your* value on breastmilk as food and breastfeeding as a means of mothering is very important, as is sharing what you discover with the professionals who you choose to support you in meeting your breastfeeding and lactation goals.

> *I still tear up over it. I know that it is kind of weird, but it is almost like a part of me died when I realized that I could not give my baby the best of what she needed.*

You might decide that you consider other aspects of mothering more important than nurturing your baby at your breasts—and that your efforts to breastfeed your baby are impeding those other aspects of mothering. You might decide that, after evaluating your family's situation, you don't think minimizing your baby's exposure to breastmilk substitutes is going to be worth the effort you'd have to expend in that process, perhaps at the expense of taking good nutritional care of yourself and the rest of your family. When you take the time to really evaluate your personal priorities and goals, you may feel less reason to defend your choices or to educate those who seem to be attacking them.

Responding to Criticism

There may be situations where you do feel like you need to respond, either to a family member, friend, health care professional, or a stranger on social media. First and foremost, being able to identify the emotions that are triggering your desire to respond is necessary. Are you angry? At whom? Are you sad? Why? Next, what do you hope to accomplish with your response? Do you want to change the mind of the person or agency that shared the message that bothered you? Who is this person? How important and on what basis is your relationship with him or her? Is the message intended to be critical, or does your experience color your perception of it? If you respond, will you provide education or awareness of something the messenger doesn't already have, or are you *seeking validation* that your experience was real and that you did the best you could? If the answer to this last question is yes or even maybe, seriously consider whether a response is worth your time and energy, and go back to when you prioritized your values with regard to motherhood and infant feeding.

You don't need validation of your experience because you already carefully considered what was best for your family and made your choice accordingly. If you find you're feeling guilt instead of regret for how breastfeeding happened (or didn't) for you, examine why you are feeling that way and see if that influences your desire to respond.

Response Techniques and Strategies

If, after honestly evaluating your motivation for responding to critical or insensitive messages, you really think doing so is a good idea, there are some strategies you can employ to help you maintain your sanity (correcting all the wrong people on the Internet can be crazy-making) and ensure that your response will be clear and received as you intended. When my children were young, I learned a lot about responding to criticism for my parenting choices at my local La Leche League meetings. I have included my favorite article by Marianne Vakiener about this topic in the Resource Chapter.

Formula companies do their best to make mothers who can physiologically provide enough breastmilk for their babes feel like they can't. They want to see full milk supplies go down to partial, so that the difference is made up with their product—for their profit.

This is a huge part of why the breastfeeding community, in general, has this "Every woman can breastfeed" idealism. Because the fact is that, in truth, the vast majority of women can. But formula companies, and their "gang" (pediatricians, pregnancy magazines, TV networks, etc.) bend and twist the truth, just enough to make moms feel insecure. Then combine that with inadequate support, and there is an epidemic of mothers who do not need to supplement, but they think that they do.

And this is why those of us with true, legitimate milk-supply issues get left, and made to feel like crap. The ones who shout, "Every woman can breastfeed! Trust your body!" are legitimately trying to help those full-supply moms who have been tricked and lied to. They are trying to save them from a version of the heartache that we endure on a daily basis. They are just completely ignorant of those of us who cannot do it on our own. We are much smaller in number, so we're not as visible to them.

It makes us supplementing moms look like we just got duped by the formula companies, because a lot of supplementing moms out there actually were. Without actually seeing what we go through on a daily basis, sacrificing virtually everything to squeeze out every last drop of milk, they can't possibly have any idea.

Originally, formula was just used for mothers who legitimately could not make enough milk, or if mother and baby were separated. Formula was created as a life-saving product. But once serious money and greed entered the equation, it became an incentive for these companies to trick mothers, and lie to them about their bodies.

Supplementation saved my daughter's life. It is a necessary and good thing for many of us, because our babies NEED to be fed. But the formula companies screw us over just as much as they do the mothers they deceive, because it makes us look like we are ignorant about breastfeeding. Which is absolutely not the truth.

Whenever I get really upset or frustrated with comments like that, I try to jump in and just educate.

—Bekki, Red Hook, NY

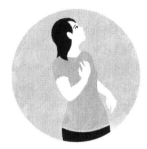

Chapter 7

If You Are Supporting a Mother with IGT

Professionals who work with breastfeeding mothers are often perplexed when they encounter a mother who claims that she can't make enough breastmilk to exclusively sustain her baby. Can't all women breastfeed? If she can gestate, can't she lactate? How would the human race have persisted if lactation could fail? We wonder whether the mother "tried hard enough," got the right support, or just didn't really want to breastfeed in the first place.

> *I hate that my midwife gives me a blank stare when I bring it up. This is something ALL medical professionals that deal with pregnant women should know about.*

> *I have fought for everything I wanted and lost which has set me up to feel discouraged about feeding my second baby.*

The mothers wonder the same things about themselves when we can't—or won't—support their efforts to breastfeed. When the "breastfeeding authorities" that mothers seek help from, be they physicians, midwives, nurses, IBCLCs, or other breastfeeding supporters (paid or volunteer) fail to acknowledge that *milk may not come* even if the mother's breasts are large, a downward spiral of anger, shame, and insecurity can overtake a mother at the very time when she least needs to feel those emotions: she is adjusting to her new role as the mother of a precious new baby.

Yet, these situations don't seem to improve even with our competent, knowledgeable support. Endeavoring to get enough milk from breasts with IGT can feel as futile as squeezing blood from a stone.

*It is a heartbreaking thing to discover during a time (postpartum)
when you are already very fragile. I had to focus on the little goals
and the time with my baby. Having a medical professional tell you
that you just need to try harder is the worst feeling in the world.
You just have to push through, never give up, and in the end be
satisfied that you did everything you could to provide as much
as you could for as long as you could.*

Breastfeeding or Lactating?

As much as we would all love to see every baby fed with exclusively
breastmilk for the first 6 months of life, when that's not possible
because of physiological or social reasons, we can support mothers
in partially breastfeeding or partially lactating. We don't often have
occasion to differentiate between the two behaviors, but separating
breastfeeding from *lactation* is one valuable approach that we can
take in our support of mothers who are unable to feed their babies
exclusively with their milk.

After suboptimal breastfeeding management (such as scheduling
feeds or limiting time at the breast); tongue tie or other issues of the
baby's oral anatomy; hormonal imbalances, like thyroid dysregulation; and other, more common (and more fixable) causes of low milk
output have been ruled out, we need to provide outstanding counseling to the mother who sought to breastfeed but cannot. Asking
her, "What about breastfeeding were you most excited about?" is
a wonderful conversation starter.

We already know that breastmilk is the superior food for babies.
Emerging research is showing us that being fed at the breast is also

important for appropriate growth and development. Most mothers fall somewhere along a continuum that looks like this:

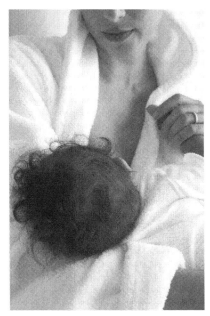 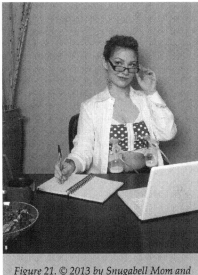

Figure 21. © 2013 by Snugabell Mom and Baby Gear. Reprinted with permission.

Breastfeeding/Closeness------Lactating/Milk

Helping a mother determine where she falls along that continuum is vital as you design the care plan that will best help her reach her breastfeeding goals. Notice the emphasis on the *mother's* goals: she will be most receptive and likely to succeed at giving her baby *her best* if we let her determine where to focus her efforts.

Keeping a baby interested in a breast that doesn't readily provide satisfaction takes work. Increasing milk output with expressing, herbs, medications, or diet also requires a commitment. There are mothers who have the desire and support to devote 100% to both efforts, but most will find that prioritizing one over the other permits the greatest chance for success.

In our New York Medical College School of Health Sciences and Practice 2013 study of mothers who experienced low milk output due to suspected or confirmed IGT, Penny Liberatos and I asked over 1,200 respondents to rate, on a scale of 1 *(very disinterested)* to 5 *(very interested)* how interested they were in building their milk supply so that they could produce as much milk as possible. Their answers indicated that most of the mothers (but not all) were very interested in taking measures to increase their milk output. We also asked the respondents to rate, on the same scale, their interest in making sure that their babies could feed at their breasts, even if they were supplementing with something other than their own milk.

More than 85% of respondents rated their interest in making more milk a 4 or a 5; about 8% of them were less interested (1 or a 2) in building their milk supplies. Just over 60% indicated high (4 or 5) interest in keeping their babies at their breasts; just over a quarter were less interested (1 or 2) in taking measures to keep their babies at their breasts. Obviously, most of those mothers felt that both aspects of the breastfeeding experience were of utmost importance. We as practitioners cannot presume to know how an individual mother feels unless we ask what about breastfeeding is *most important to her.*

It is vital to keep in mind, as well, a mother's feelings about breastfeeding and lactation may shift or change as she begins working on the care plan that has been developed for her unique circumstance. She may discover that a regime of pumping and taking supplements feels more intrusive than helpful or that the learning curve of coaxing her baby back to her not-so-milky breast is steeper than she thought it would be and her feelings of rejection—even though *we* know that her baby loves and needs her—are painfully real in those moments.

As breastfeeding supporters, follow-up with all of the mothers that we help is expected. With IGT moms, follow-up needs to occur *sooner and more frequently.* The most important message that we can communicate to a mother is that we want to support her in meeting *her* breastfeeding goals, even if those goals change or shift. Continually ask each mother what she hopes for. Educate her about what, in your experience, might be realistic for her to expect from her body. Give her the tools she needs to make breastfeeding work in the manner that best satisfies what she's seeking from the experience.

Support When Milk Is the Priority

Many mothers, when asked what they were most looking forward to about breastfeeding, talk about the milk—the nutrition, immune properties, and digestibility that make human milk the superior food for human babies.

I've had countless mothers and breastfeeding supporters ask me how to help a mother make more milk. Which herb works best? At what dose? Does oatmeal help improve milk output? What about beer? Do I recommend medications? As an IBCLC who is not also an herbalist, nutritionist, nurse practitioner, midwife, or physician, my scope of practice is limited. I do not feel qualified to discuss or prescribe specific herbs, foods, or medications with an individual mother. However, I am happy to refer her to professionals in my community and resources that can answer her specific questions and to share general information about ways to increase milk output. My favorite information sources on these topics are listed in the Resource Chapter. I can also tell her what I've seen work for the mothers with histories that are similar to hers, so that she has a starting point from which to communicate with the appropriate health care professionals.

One caution that I freely offer, however, is to match the galactagogue to the underlying cause of low milk output. This means that a thorough history into what might be affecting the mother's ability to make milk needs to be taken, and a thorough knowledge of how the available galactagogues work in a mother's body must be applied. Suggesting that a mother "try fenugreek" because that has worked for other mothers or recommending the latest hot herb blend on the market without satisfying these two foundational requirements can be expensive to the mother, both financially and to her own health. Some galactagogues can actually make milk production worse if they are given to mothers with other underlying hormonal complications.

Determining which galactagogue will be "most effective" is difficult because every lactation problem is unique. Our study found that most of the commonly recommended galactagogues did not have a substantial effect on milk output.

This cannot be stated or emphasized enough: in any situation where milk output is questioned, the most important thing to assess and correct, if necessary, is milk transfer. If milk is not being removed from the breast efficiently enough (such as if baby is unable to latch properly and do the work of removing milk) or often enough (such as when pacifiers are being used to space out feedings or when parents are attempting to put their baby on a feeding schedule), milk production can suffer. *Be sure to rule out problems of breastfeeding management and infant anatomy before concluding that the problem of milk output is due to the anatomy or physiology of the mother.*

In addition, while hormonal issues in the mother may be related to IGT, they are not, in and of themselves, *the same* as IGT. A mother can have IGT without accompanying endocrinopathy. Conversely, a mother can have problems with her thyroid, androgens, insulin, or other hormones without also having an insufficient complement of glandular tissue.

Hormonal issues and IGT are often but not always comorbid. Referral to a competent endocrinologist, perhaps one who specializes in reproductive endocrinology and is *knowledgeable about the endocrinology of lactation* may be necessary for the mother with a complex hormonal history. An outstanding resource for assessing all of the various complications that can affect breastmilk output is *The Breastfeeding Mother's Guide to Making More Milk,* by Diana West and Lisa Marasco (2008).

In terms of milk transfer, ankyloglossia (tongue tie), and/or restriction of the upper labial frenulum (lip tie), can affect a baby's ability to latch properly to the breast and remove milk. Mothers who experienced breast changes in pregnancy and who seemed to have enough milk for 2 or more weeks postpartum before struggling with milk production are more likely to have a tongue tied baby than IGT.

Of course, it is possible that a mother with IGT could have a baby with anatomical restrictions creating the "perfect storm" of lactation difficulty. If you are unsure you can recognize or assess for the four types of tongue tie and there are no professionals in your community who have this skill, there are helpful resources online. I've listed them in the resource section of this book, along with additional, in-depth information sources about milk supply issues due to infant problems with milk transfer. I have seen far too many mothers believe that their milk supply problems are inherent to their own bodies when the more likely answer was a missed tongue tie or lip tie that precluded effective milk transfer and breast emptying.

It is important to remember that *you don't have to be the breastfeeding expert* if that's not your area of focus or practice. Identify and refer to the peer support organizations (such as La Leche League) in your community and to the professional lactation consultants (IBCLCs) in your area. While mothers appreciate an ob–gyn or a pediatrician who is supportive of breastfeeding, they are most thankful for health care professionals who can recognize when it's time to direct a mother to another resource. Just as you would refer to a cardiologist when you suspect a complex issue of the heart or to an ear, nose, and throat doctor when a baby has recurrent, unexplained ear infections, do not hesitate to refer your patients with complex infant feeding issues to an IBCLC and to collaborate with her on care plans and courses of action. When you've established that a mother truly has a milk-making issue that *she wants to devote herself to overcoming,* the following solutions may come to mind.

Pumping and Hand-Expression of Milk

See Chapter 5, Feeding Your Baby, for information about pumping and hand-expressing milk to improve milk supply.

Herbal Galactagogues

Because of their availability, relative safety, and long history of use in traditional societies, herbs are a common go-to when a mother wants to increase her milk supply. Herbal galactagogues may be helpful for both improving the potential of the breast tissue that a mother has and normalizing her hormone set (usually her blood sugar and insulin sensitivity).

Although there are many anecdotal and clinical reports of herbs, such as fenugreek, goat's rue, moringa oleifera, and shatavari improving the milk supplies of mothers, even dramatically in some cases, there is still insufficient evidence, such as that obtained in a clinical trial, for their safety and efficacy (Forinash, Yancey, Barnes, & Myles, 2012; Zapantis, Steinberg, & Schilit, 2012). A systematic review of studies, including those that demonstrated galactagogue efficacy, was conducted by Mortel and Mehta (2013). These authors also concluded that further evidence is necessary before recommendation of herbal galactagogues should be undertaken. The major weaknesses found in the existing literature include a lack of randomization, controls, or blinding; small sample sizes; high dropout rates; and failure to optimize breastfeeding management and milk removal (Academy of Breastfeeding Medicine, 2011a).

It is important to consider, as well, that results obtained after study of lactating women with a full complement of glandular tissue may or may not be generalizable to women with IGT. Do certain herbs work differently in one physiological environment than in another? Would the increase in milk production be statistically significant if the milk volumes being studied were smaller (not a full supply) to begin with?

Research on women with low milk output due to suspected IGT—when all other possible reasons for the deficiency have been ruled out—is absolutely necessary. I appreciate the difficulty in performing such research: difficulty in standardizing herbal dosages, the logistical obstacles involved in uniform milk collection and output measurement techniques, and the need to study only those mothers who are exclusively expressing milk by pump—so as not to pose an ethical issue by taking a baby off his mother's breast—are all problems that would need to be overcome in the search for an aptly sized sample and pristine data collection methods.

Does this mean we should discourage mothers from trying herbs for boosting milk production? No. If the mother's full history is understood and the herb or herbs are matched to her unique situation, there may be some benefit. Some professionals have suggested that a placebo effect exists in some mothers; if milk output is improved without risk to the mother or her baby, why not go with it?

Drugs to Increase Milk Output

There is some evidence to support the use of certain drugs for the improvement of milk output in lactating mothers. These drugs were formulated for gastrointestinal issues but offer the side effect of causing lactation in those who use them.

Ingram, Taylor, Churchill, Pike, and Greenwood (2012) studied the effect of metoclopramide (Reglan) and domperidone (sold under several names) on the breastmilk output of mothers with premature babies in the neonatal intensive care unit, and found that both drugs significantly increased the amount of milk that the mothers were able to produce in a 10-day period.

While this study offers some evidence for the use of these drugs to improve milk output, before I wholeheartedly jump to universal recommendations for all women with low milk supply, I'd like to see a similar blinded, randomized controlled trial that includes a placebo group that receives no intervention, since the milk output of a mother of a premature baby may naturally increase dramatically as the mother's original due date approaches. Fife et al. (2011) offered this type of study for metoclopramide and found that milk output did increase in both groups but not statistically significantly enough in the treatment group to be attributable to the drug. I'd also like to see a sufficiently large sample of mothers *with IGT* before I rule in—or out—the efficacy of drugs to help with milk production after a healthy, full-term baby is born.

> *Domperidone literally saved my breastfeeding relationship with all four of my children. I went from producing 7 oz a day to 20 oz on 180 mg of domperidone. It is legal in Canada, which is wonderful, but it's not available in the U.S. Many mothers go without this miracle drug and it would be amazing if this could be changed.*

Clinically, I have seen domperidone improve the milk output of several women with suspected or confirmed IGT, most of them with BMI of greater than 25 or greater than 29.9 ("overweight" or "obese"). I attribute this improvement to the ability of domperidone, a dopamine antagonist, to keep prolactin levels at a sustained, higher concentration in the bloodstream. This may be helpful for mothers whose breasts, for whatever reasons (insufficient glandular tissue upon which prolactin receptors can reside and an obesity-induced hormonal milieu that prevents the early establishment of prolactin receptors are two that come to mind), did not experience the manufacture of prolactin receptors (see Chapter 4 for details about lactation complications in mothers with higher BMIs or insulin-resistant mothers).

Given that early and frequent suckling is necessary for the development of these receptors within the glandular tissue of the breasts (de Carvalho, Robertson, Friedman, & Klaus, 1983), it makes sense that, in mothers with less glandular tissue, fewer receptors will ultimately be present, even under the most favorable early breastfeeding conditions. Domperidone may help ensure that circulating prolactin has enough time to be received by those receptors, even if they are fewer in number, and thus enable a higher milk output from the existing glandular tissue. While metoclopramide, also a dopamine antagonist, can accomplish this, it is less favored for long-term milk production assistance because of the fact that, unlike domperidone, metoclopramide crosses the blood–brain barrier, which can result in extreme depression and anxiety in mothers who use it. Because mothers who are struggling with breastfeeding seem to be already at increased risk for perinatal mood disorders

(Watkins, Meltzer-Brody, Zolnoun, & Stuebe, 2011), my clinical instinct leads me to counsel mothers to avoid using this drug at all costs.

I don't believe that improving breastmilk output or optimizing the breastfeeding experience of any mother is worth risking her overall health, and the risk inherent with metoclopramide use seems greater than the potential benefit.

Unfortunately, in the United States, metoclopramide is "more prescribable," in that there are no regulations in place to prevent its sale, either for its intended purpose (to slow gastric emptying) or for off-label purposes, such as is done with domperidone. There are no controversies (other than the "off-label" use) around domperidone in other countries, but in the United States, the legal status of the drug remains in flux as of this writing.

Currently, domperidone has "orphan" drug status. According to the U.S. Food and Drug Administration, the Orphan Drug Designation program provides orphan status to drugs and biologics, which are defined as those intended for the safe and effective treatment, diagnosis, or prevention of rare diseases/disorders that affect fewer than 200,000 people in the United States, or that affect more than 200,000 persons but for which the costs of developing and marketing a treatment drug are not expected to be recovered.

Perhaps after efficacy and safety for mothers with lactation difficulties and their babies can be more conclusively supported by research, domperidone will be a more readily accepted treatment for augmenting milk production. Until then, there are compounding pharmacies that will make domperidone available with a valid prescription from a health care provider with prescribing power.

In addition, mothers may order the drug from overseas pharmacies but may run a legal risk in doing so if they do not have a physician's prescription. *Any discussion of domperidone with mothers should include information about this legal risk.*

Finally, it is important to remember that there will be some drugs that can actually decrease a mother's milk supply. These include antihistamines, birth control pills, and other drugs that interact with the endocrine system, such as clomid.

Drugs for Other Uses in the Breastfeeding/ Lactating Mother

The role of medications in the breastfeeding mother is commonly misunderstood, with many health care professionals believing (and counseling their patients) that medications are unsafe to use.

It is important to recognize that pregnancy and lactation, while closely related, are two different periods in a woman's life, and a drug that is contraindicated in pregnancy is not necessarily unsafe to baby or mother during lactation. In fact, there are drugs that, if used appropriately during pregnancy and lactation, may improve a mother's ability to breastfeed her baby.

As a health care professional, you will be a preferred resource for helping a mother weigh any possible risks of using a medication against its potential benefits. In lactation, the greater risk is typically the mediation's possible effect on milk supply, *not* whether or how much of the medication passes from the mother into the baby via the breastmilk.

Two comprehensive resources, The National Institute of Health's LactMed and Dr. Thomas Hale's InfantRisk Center (as well as his 2012 book, *Medications and Mothers' Milk*), present evidence-based information on thousands of medications, covering such aspects as the half-life, molecular size (which affects whether the medication can even pass into the breast alveoli), age of the nursing baby, and amount of the maternal dose that may be received by the baby. All of these factors can figure into a practitioner's decision whether to prescribe or recommend a medication. See the Resource Chapter for links to these and other resources.

Endocrinology and Lactation

One area of medicine that seems to have a close relationship to lactation is endocrinology. Research to more accurately determine reference ranges for particular hormones during lactation is limited, but widespread clinical experience indicates that lactation issues are common among women with hormonal problems. Marasco et al. (2000) presented a series of three cases of endocrinopathy that were correlated with low milk production and may also have had something to do with glandular development.

It is sensible to consider that if a mother needs medication or a diet change to normalize her hormones (either to get and/or stay pregnant or just to feel good in day-to-day life), medication or a change in her diet may be helpful to her during lactation as well, especially if there are breastfeeding problems that seem to be traceable to maternal anatomy or physiology.

Metformin and synthroid are two medications that come to mind. Consider also that the hormones that are suppressed during lactation (for example, estrogen and progesterone) *should remain suppressed* when trying to augment a mother's milk output. For this reason, any birth control, estrogen therapy (to treat vaginal dryness or migraines, for example), or other medication that introduces hormones that are naturally suppressed in lactation should be carefully evaluated in any breastfeeding mother, but particularly for the mother who is struggling with low milk supply.

> *Unfortunately, I experienced much confusion and shame about both my breasts and inability to produce milk for my babies.*
>
> *I have harbored guilt, disappointment, and anger about this for years. I confronted my OB/GYN with my research six months ago, and she agreed that I have IGT.*
>
> *When I said it angers me that no one "warned" me that breastfeeding might not be possible with either of my children despite the appearance of my breasts, having severe PCOS, and zero changes during or after my pregnancies, she replied that it would only discourage mothers from trying to breast feed. I feel so frustrated with all of this.*

Foods to Increase Milk Output

While the scientific literature is lacking in this area, there have been reports of women in traditional societies and clinical observations of mothers using certain foods, such as sesame seeds, oats, and brewer's yeast, to improve their milk output. In addition, other foods have been recognized as anti-lactogenic and should be avoided. These include mint, sage, and, in some cases, caffeine, which may also include chocolate. See the Resource Chapter for more information about foods as galactagogues.

As a health care provider, your best bet when a mother asks you about foods to improve her milk supply will be to point her in the direction of evidence that supports or doesn't support robust lactation. Much of this evidence will come from traditional societies and the clinical observations of those who work most closely with mothers and their babies. As with herbal galactagogues, try not to be too quick to dismiss a mother's report that something she is eating is helping her milk supply. Even if she is experiencing a placebo effect, the feeling that she has some influence over her ability to produce milk may be the difference between keeping at it and giving up sooner than she wanted to.

One more important concept concerning diet and breastmilk production is covered in greater depth in the chapter on hormones and glandular development: the effect of macronutrient content in an overall diet on milk output. While the scientific literature doesn't tell us directly that a low-glycemic, protein-rich diet may improve lactation outcomes, our emerging understanding of the relationship between insulin sensitivity and milk production (Lemay et al., 2013) may lead us to the conclusion that a daily diet and activity regimen that normalizes a mother's production and uptake of insulin may also improve milk output.

It is still unclear whether improving insulin sensitivity during the postpartum period may make up for deficiencies in glandular development during puberty and pregnancy, but in my opinion, measures taken to improve a mother's overall health (such as weight loss and correction of factors that may lead to metabolic disease later in life) are well worth trying, whether they immediately improve milk output or not. Clinically, I have seen mothers make these dietary adjustments and initially see a slight dip in their milk output. Those who stick with the changes for a few more days have seen a significant rebound and improvement in their milk supplies after about 2 weeks.

Donor Human Milk

It makes sense that when a mother values human milk as the optimal food for her baby but is unable to produce the amount that is needed to sustain him, she may consider obtaining, per the guidance of the WHO's *Global Strategy for Infant and Young Child Feeding* (WHO, 2003), the next best thing for her baby: donor breastmilk from another human mother.

There are two sources for acquiring donor milk: via a milk bank or "informally," through a mother-to-mother milk sharing arrangement. While the former does occur, it is more commonly practiced in the hospital or when the baby is under a month old. Banked donor milk can be expensive (testing, administration of the milk banks, and processing are costly) and is available by prescription, usually for those babies who would not survive or thrive if fed breastmilk substitutes.

Mother-to-mother milk sharing is a practice that is taking place at an increasing rate in many communities. In our 2013 study of mothers with low milk output due to suspected or confirmed IGT, Penny Liberatos and I found that 26.8% (n = 857) of respondents had used donor milk obtained in a milk sharing arrangement to supplement their own milk supplies. As a health care provider, you may have strong, perhaps negative feelings about this method of supplementation because of your concerns over disease transmission, hygiene, or your personal experiences with commercially prepared breastmilk substitutes.

These concerns were addressed in depth by Gribble and Hausman (2012), and are summarized in Chapter 5 in this book. Informing yourself about the comparative risks between any two feeding methods so that you can properly counsel mothers and help them evaluate and mitigate those risks that are unique to their situations may become an important part of your practice, if it has not already. The resources that were shared in the aforementioned chapter also include specific tests and health-related questions that might be prudent for a mother to ask of her potential milk donors. You may find yourself in a position to counsel a woman who wants to be a milk donor and needs screening blood work to give to her recipient family, or you may be asked about accepting milk from another breastfeeding mother by a family with milk supply problems. Familiarize yourself with the real risks and benefits of the practice in a variety of environments and circumstances so that you are truly ready to offer evidence-based information about the use of donor human breastmilk.

In your support of families that choose to acquire donor breastmilk and feed it to their babies, you will need to consider the potential ramifications of "brokering" that milk—of connecting a mother in need with a mother who has milk to share. As an IBCLC, I *do not, under any circumstances* serve as a broker between mothers because I do not have access to the full health history of either the donor or the infant/child that will receive the milk. Unless you, in your scope of practice, have access to the blood work, lifestyle considerations, medications, and other relevant information (and few of us do) for both the *donor* and *recipient*, you may also not be in a position to broker breastmilk. You can, however, inform both donors and mothers in need about milk sharing organizations online, mothers' groups in the community where milk may be shared between mothers who meet and get to know each other, and most importantly, about how a recipient mother can carefully and actively screen any potential donors.

At the very least, the following are red flags:

- The donor mother refuses to provide answers to health questions, such as drug (prescription or recreational) use, smoking, sexual behavior, or blood test results of interest.

- The donor mother is not actually feeding her child, and she is lactating for another reason (an important exception to this may be the mother of an infant who has recently died; in this case, the opportunity to share the milk she has may be a welcome step in coping with her loss).

• The milk is being offered for sale rather than as a donation. In many U.S. states, the sale of human tissue, which breastmilk is, is illegal. In other states, this practice is perfectly within the limits of the law. It is feasible for recipients to pay for blood work, milk storage bags/containers, any shipping costs, or other expenses incidental to the expression, storage, and delivery of the milk, but milk selling may be an indicator of behavior that presents additional risk to the recipient family.

The use of donor breastmilk has been a step toward healing and reconciliation with their own bodies for many mothers with IGT. Being able to provide accurate, evidence-based information about the risks and benefits will be crucial to your ability to support a mother who wants to make this choice. An excellent commentary on being a professional in support of milk-sharing mothers can be found at *http://www.ambermccann.com/blog/milksharing.*

Support When Breastfeeding—Feeding at the Breast—Is the Goal

There are mothers who feel more strongly about *how* they feed their babies than *what* is being fed. When asked what they were most looking forward to about breastfeeding, these mothers will answer that they value the closeness, bonding, and mother–baby relationship that is built into breastfeeding.

Yes, a breastfeeding mother can engage in behaviors that divert her attention away from her baby, or her experience of breastfeeding may be so unpleasant that feeding at the breast really *isn't* most conducive to the exchange of love that the physiology of prolactin and oxytocin so beautifully facilitate for most breastfeeding mothers.

> *If you want the nursing relationship, do not listen to those who tell you to stop. It is very much worth fighting for.*

Conversely, a bottle-feeding mother can learn to employ positioning, skin-to-skin contact, and specific bottle-feeding practices to more closely approximate what a breastfeeding dyad experiences together. In this section, I assume that the mother you are supporting values keeping her baby at her breast and has made the choice to take measures to accomplish that—that she *values breastfeeding as more than a method of delivering food to her baby.* It is important to remember that for some mothers, this is not the case. The only way to know what a mother wants from her breastfeeding relationship is to *engage in a continuing dialogue with her about it.*

The challenge for some mother–baby pairs when there is insufficient milk production to exclusively breastfeed is keeping the baby interested in feeding—or merely being—at his mother's breast. Several factors may affect their ability to nurse at the breast, and these are discussed in the following sections.

The Baby's Age

Younger babies who have not been away from the breast very much yet may be more able to instinctively root for their mothers' breasts and find comfort there, if not also nutritional sustenance. Skin-to-skin contact allows mother and baby to experience each other with more senses and can help protect the baby's instinctual tendencies toward his mother. Keeping baby dressed lightly and keeping mom in an open button-down shirt allows them to relax with the baby between his mother's breasts. He can hear her heart beating, smell her milk, and feel her warmth. If mom has to be up and about, perhaps to take care of older siblings, a soft, wrap-style sling can allow this skin-to-skin contact while her hands are free.

How Much Milk the Mother Actually Makes

Some mothers with IGT find that they can produce and store enough milk for an entire feeding, but they struggle to keep up with the number of feedings per day that their babies need. These mothers don't have to supplement very much because they are producing 2–3 ounces at a time, just not the full volume of milk their babies need to thrive, even with more frequent breastfeeding or expressing. When these babies are brought to their mothers' breasts, there is milk there.

Other mothers find that they are only able to produce a fraction of what their babies need at each feeding and need to offer supplementation throughout the day in order to keep their babies adequately fed. For these pairs, efforts to help the baby associate satiety with being at the breast can be very helpful.

The use of an at-breast supplementing tool so that the baby gets his nourishment while suckling at his mother's breast can be a wonderful technique, and it also serves to protect the mother's milk supply because most, if not all, feedings will still be offered at the breast. It is vital, however, that *any sucking problems on the baby's side are recognized and resolved before the introduction of at-breast supple-mentation.* If a baby is unable to efficiently and properly remove the milk that is there in his mother's breast, the addition of a tube feeder to the scenario may only worsen it. Babies are wonderfully intelligent and adaptive; they will do what they need to do to feed themselves, and they will protest when they have to work harder than they know they have to. This leads to the next factor in keeping a baby interested in his mother's breast.

How Baby Has Been Fed up to This Point

While improvements are continually being made in the quality and availability of competent breastfeeding support, there are still mothers and babies who want to breastfeed but are victimized by gross misunderstandings of normal newborn behavior and how lactation works.

Poor or absent breastfeeding support in the immediate post-partum time can create difficulty for any mother, but for mothers with IGT, these missteps in getting breastfeeding started can be nearly impossible to recover from because of the physiological deficits that these mothers may have (see Chapter 4 for more infor-mation about the role of physiology in lactation with IGT).

The most damaging practice to the establishment of breastfeeding that I see is too-early supplementation with too much supplement, using a "too-easy" feeding vessel. *Please do not confuse this with ill-informed guidance to not offer supplementation to a hungry baby.* I am speaking specifically about the offering bottles of breast-milk substitute to babies in the first 72 hours of life when weight loss has not approached 10% of birth weight, after adjustment for maternal IV fluids that may have been taken on by the baby during the labor and delivery, which may artificially inflate the birthweight (Chantry, Nommsen-Rivers, Peerson, Cohen, & Dewey, 2011; Noel-Weiss, Woodend, Peterson, Gibb, & Groll, 2011). The Academy of Breastfeeding Medicine, in its Clinical Protocol #3: *Hospital Guidelines for the Use of Supplementary Feedings in the Healthy Term Breastfed Neonate* (2009), *(http://www.bfmed.org/Media/Files/Protocols/ Protocol%203%20English%20Supplementation.pdf)*, presents commonly ignored contraindications to the supplementation of a new baby and stressed that "reasons for supplementation in term, healthy infants are few" (p. 176).

Even when IGT is a problem, supplementation is very rarely indicated before the mother's milk would have come in anyway (2–3 days after the birth or longer after a surgical delivery or in mothers with a prepregnant BMI of greater than 29.9). In widespread clinical experience, the production of colostrum seems to be less dependent on the presence or amount of glandular tissue or on any hormonal problems a mother may have that interfere with lactation. Once again, this assumes that the baby does not have an anatomical challenge, such as ankyloglossia, that impedes his ability to suck properly and stimulate the transfer of food from the breast. Always assess (or find someone who can competently assess) the infant's sucking ability before developing a care plan for a dyad.

However, after the first few days, supplementation may truly be necessary for the IGT mother–baby pair. How the supplement is given can be detrimental to breastfeeding, or it can be supportive and conducive to preserving a baby's normal instincts. In the first 2 weeks, when we are still watching and waiting to see what a mother's milk production capacity might be, offering supplements via cup (such as those flexible, plastic cups given with cough syrup), eyedropper, or syringe (pointed at the baby's cheek and slowly discharged into the baby's mouth) may be preferred in the short term to offering a bottle, since these methods demand little participation from the baby and enable him to spend his energy on what breastfeeding he is able to do.

> *Being able to breastfeed at all really helped my self-esteem. With extremely small breasts and nipples, I doubted my femininity, but being able to supply my babies' milk, even by nursing very often, boosted my morale as a woman as well as a mother.*

Another method of short-term, early supplementation that may be protective of breastfeeding is finger-feeding: the use of a small tube attached to a supply of the supplement of choice and taped to a clean finger that is inserted into the baby's mouth. A finger-feeder is best used in cases where the baby needs a little suck training, perhaps after tongue tie revision or if his suck was compromised during the birth process or was due to another congenital issue of his oral structure. For more detailed information about finger-feeding, see the device that Dr. Alison Hazelbaker designed for this purpose at *http://fingerfeeder.com/index.html.*

When Bottle-Feeding Is Necessary

Once it becomes clear that a mother will be unable to exclusively breastfeed her baby because of insufficient milk production, if she is unable or unwilling to supplement feedings at the breast, there are specific bottle-feeding techniques that can be supportive of and more physiologically like breastfeeding. The Resource Chapter at the end of this book provides a list of specific books, articles, and handouts that provide information about how to bottle-feed in a manner that helps to protect the breastfeeding relationship between a mother and baby.

> You can still breastfeed. I have recently been introduced to a group of moms and many of them are giving up or exclusively pumping. I pumped, but I nursed. I think you can become bitter and hate nursing moms.
>
> There is no reason to think this way. You can breastfeed. I have for 17 months. My son is eating foods and he still nurses. I had to supplement, but I did at the breast. On occasion, he received a bottle, but only fed a certain way. I think you can complain or you can learn and fight for what you want. It doesn't have to be all or nothing.

Make the Breast an Appealing Destination

If the baby is more than a few weeks old, has been aggressively bottle-fed, or has had repeated unpleasant experiences at the breast, the road to restoring the breast as the biologically normal place for comfort and, perhaps, nourishment may be a long one. The most important thing to remember—and to encourage families to remember—is that the breast needs to be a nice place for the baby to be. Warm baths together, skin-to-skin contact, and the ability to relax together, perhaps with a little no-expectations suckling at the breast will be helpful steps toward facilitating mother–baby communication at the breast.

The process of enticing a baby back to his mother's breast will take time and can be especially frustrating for a mother who feels rejected or like her baby doesn't like her. Reassuring a mother that she is absolutely her baby's favorite person in the world and helping her to emotionally separate lactation from breastfeeding, even if only at first, are important elements of the support you will offer. Although it is heartbreaking to have to be in the position of choosing between breastfeeding and lactation, mothers who opt to invest energy into keeping their babies at their breasts are rewarded richly for their patience and perseverance when their babies finally "get it."

Perhaps the greatest victory for a mother who works to keep her baby feeding at her breasts comes after he has reached toddlerhood and is ready to receive the majority of his nutrition from appropriate solid foods. If there is even a small supply of milk available, breastfeeding a child past the age of 12 months continues to confer nutritional and immunological advantages (Dewey, 2001; Goldman, Goldblum, & Garza, 1983). However, the ability to continue to offer comfort and closeness through the ups and downs of toddler life (and perhaps beyond) is a prize many breastfeeding mothers are so happy to have.

> At present my baby boy is weaning me gently at 35.25 months old. It's been a slow and lovely, yet heartbreaking process for me. I dream that one day I could exclusively breastfeed, but this is likely my last nursing experience. It's been amazing and I'm so blessed that I found the SNS and support aside from the lack that was being presented to me. I can't imagine not having had this experience with my child and feel sad that I was sabotaged by

*doctors and nurses with my oldest son. I pray that every woman
has the opportunity to experience nursing their child if even by
unconventional standards.*

When a Mother Is Truly Committed to Increasing Her Milk Output and Feeding at Her Breast

There will be some mothers who have the time, resources, support, and inclination to devote to truly maximizing both their milk-making potential and the practice of keeping their babies at their breasts. For some of these mothers, milk production is already high, or their babies are already naturally attached to comfort nursing; your job will be easy with these mothers.

Unfortunately, for most mothers, the success curve for accomplishing both goals may be steep. For this reason, it is important to *continually reassess* how a mother feels about both breastfeeding and lactation. How can you do this? Ask her. Frequently! We need to provide more frequent, more diligent follow-up to our clients who are making breastfeeding/lactation work with IGT. Remind the mother that she can change her mind whenever she wants about what she's willing to do with breastfeeding. The continuum that was described earlier in this chapter is a terrific tool for communication with a mother.

Assigning numbers to each aspect of breastfeeding may provide the best measure that is reliable and valid between visits. At your first consult, a mother may state that she feels a 9 out of 10 about her commitment to making as much milk as she can (and, therefore, wants to take the time-consuming measures you may suggest to her to do this) and a 7 out of 10 about the investment in keeping her baby at her breast. A few days later, when you ask her again, this same mother may tearfully report that the endless milk expression is making her feel like she's missing out on her baby's precious fresh-baby days, but the time she spends with him at her breast is incredibly rewarding and she'd like to do whatever it takes to keep him interested there. Her new ratings are 4 out of 10 for lactation and 10 out of 10 for breastfeeding, so your care plan for her will change accordingly, and you will be transparent with her about what each behavior or technique you're asking of her is intended to accomplish.

> *I think the massage breasts/set up SNS/latch baby/breast compressions/fix latch/listen for swallowing/re-tape SNS/pump/wash pump and SNS regimen every 2–3 hours is too much for an exhausted worried new mom. Where is the support for letting mom get a good stretch of sleep once in a while?*

Keep in mind that if you do not keep the lines of communication wide open for this kind of conversation to take place, the mother, in the common effort to not let her health care provider down (that's you!), might just shut down, tell you a story of compliance that may not be true, and be one of those moms that "falls off the face of the Earth," as some tend to do, don't they?

Mothers need to know that we get how difficult this road is, and that we are here to give them the tools they need to succeed, however that success will look for them.

Developing the Care Plan

When designing or modifying a care plan for any mother, IGT or not, I make sure to communicate the following points to her and any supporters she has.

- ◆ **What I'm asking her to do.**

   Pump your breasts for 15 minutes after every feeding, at least eight times in 24 hours.

- ◆ **Why I'm asking her to do it.**

   This extra stimulation will help us to see whether your milk production problem is due to your body, your baby's ability to transfer milk well, or perhaps both.

- ◆ **How long I want her to perform the behavior.**

   I will check in with you on Friday morning, after you've done this for three days. You won't have to spend your entire life attached to the pump after that.

- ◆ **What the consequences of not performing the behavior could be.**

   I know this seems like a lot, but it's the best and fastest way we can tell what's going on…you may be tempted to skip a pumping session or not go the whole three days. That's your choice, but we'll know best what to do next if you can give this 100% for just that long.

- ◆ **How to measure the outcome of the behavior.**

   Keep a log of your feeding and pumping sessions until Friday morning. (I then draw a sample log page in a notebook or on a piece of paper that she has.)

Write down the time of day, how your baby fed, how much supplement he took, how long you pumped for, and what you got out of your breasts in that time. It's okay if you don't get much—or anything—at first or ever, just keep at it. If you experience pain, blood, anything else, call me right away and we'll figure it out.

In addition to communicating with the mother, you must ensure she has the tools she needs to carry out your recommendations. Does her pump work? Does she feel comfortable using the at-breast supplementing device without you? Is she comfortable positioning her baby at her breast? Does she know how to use and store the milk her sister is sharing from her own freezer stash?

If you are not an IBCLC (or even if you are one!), you may feel like you don't have the knowledge, time, or the resources to fully support a mother with IGT (though if you read this book, it should equip you with the information you need). This is okay! Be honest with her. She is looking to you for support and if you're unable to provide it, tell her what your limits are and where she might go in your community or otherwise to find more information and support.

To Tell or Not to Tell

Perhaps the single most controversial topic about supporting mothers with lactation insufficiency or failure is whether and how to tell them their bodies are not making enough milk to exclusively nourish their babies. As breastfeeding advocates, we may have difficulty embracing that lactation is not as stable or reliable a system as we're selling it to be, or perhaps as it once was a generation or two ago. However, with the rising rate of other, possibly related health problems, more mothers cannot simply rely on the advice to "trust their bodies" or the advice that "if you can gestate, you can lactate." Something else is going on.

The real dilemma for us as breastfeeding supporters, though, is the fear of undermining a mother's self-efficacy. There is significant literature to support this dilemma: we know well that a woman's confidence in her ability to breastfeed is a major factor in whether and how long she will actually carry out the behavior. In the informed opinion of many in our professional community, to suggest to a mother that she might have problems breastfeeding is equivalent to telling her not to even bother trying; the message that her body might not be able to do it will become a self-fulfilling prophecy.

This attitude, however, fails to consider two things: the counseling skills that are used in delivering information about potential risk factors for lactation failure, and the strength of the intention to breastfeed. Obviously, no one believes that a practitioner should examine a woman's breasts and cursorily offer something to the effect of "ooh, you might have some breastfeeding problems, see you next time." A comprehensive discussion about what, specifically, identifies this particular woman's risk factors for lactation trouble is necessary. This, of course, requires that any practitioner who works with mothers in the perinatal period be equipped with a working knowledge and understanding of how lactation works and what might affect it (examples and citations can be found in the earlier chapters of this book). It also requires very strong counseling skills and the time during the encounter to use them.

The strength of a mother's intention to breastfeed seems to be largely underestimated by members of the breastfeeding support community who feel strongly that mothers should not, under any circumstances, be told that their breasts might not function fully or properly until after lactation failure has actually occurred. It is correct that none of the risk factors discussed in this book—physical markers, obvious or subtle underdevelopment of the breasts, high BMI, endocrinopathy—are 100% predictive of lactation failure. We cannot say with any certainty that a mother will not make enough milk for her baby, even if we're dealing with a mother who struggled to produce milk for a prior baby.

Consider, however, a different health scenario. We can't say with 100% certainty that all smokers will develop cancer or other illnesses. Some smokers use tobacco throughout their entire lives and go on to die of "old age" or "natural causes" after many more years than nonsmokers, correct? Yet, we do not hesitate to educate the public that smoking is *a risk factor for*—not a guarantee of—poor health outcomes.

In recent years, clinical observation and research has given the lactation support community enough evidence and information to identify risk factors for (not guarantees of!) lactation failure that it behooves us as practitioners to share that information. Just as antismoking campaigns do not simply toss off the message, "if you smoke, you might die," without more information, it is similarly possible to tailor messages about breastfeeding risk factors such that we inform mothers rather than discourage or scare them.

However, in our study of mothers with breastfeeding difficulty, Penny Liberatos and I discovered that fewer than 20% of our respondents preferred to not be told at all, unless their milk output was low, whether their breasts had physical markers that may or may not have foreshadowed difficulty lactating. Of course, this finding was somewhat biased in that all of the respondents had actually experienced lactation failure to some degree. A survey of first-time-pregnant women about whether they'd want to be told would offer a good basis for comparison and help us determine just how profound our sample's bias was.

Additionally, we asked mothers to rate on a scale of 1 *(not at all)* to 5 *(very much)* whether learning that they would not be able to exclusively breastfeed caused them to want to "quit and exclusively bottle-feed." The results are represented in the following graph:

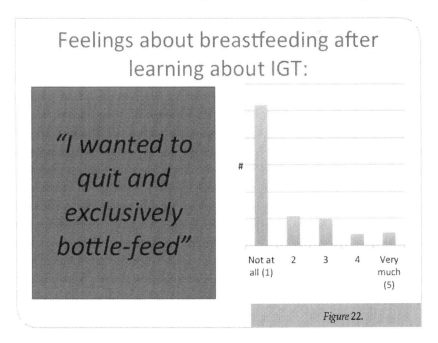

Figure 22.

Clearly, in our study population (primarily white, college-educated residents of the United States, ages 20–39), breastfeeding intention remained strong even after the realization that exclusive breastfeeding would likely be impossible. It is worth considering that populations where breastfeeding intention (perhaps measured by the local initiation rate) is not robust may require a more sensitive approach to counseling about IGT or other conditions that might affect breastfeeding, but to withhold information from mothers is not good practice. Take the time to develop your repertoire of counseling techniques and language that informs mothers without discouraging or scaring them, such as in the following manner:

Some, but certainly not all, mothers with widely spaced, asymmetrical breasts like yours have some trouble making enough milk for their babies. Here are the things we can do together to make sure your breastfeeding experience gets off to the best start, and here's what you'll need to know and observe in those first few weeks so that you know things are going well.

How wonderful would it be if every mother received such attention and follow-up care? All mothers need it, but the mother with IGT or other risk factors for lactation failure will most assuredly crash and burn without that kind of support.

Our study also examined the relationship between specific types of support and breastfeeding duration: which support factors were correlated with mothers breastfeeding longer. For this analysis, we included only those respondents who reported the intention to exclusively breastfeed for 6 months, wide breast spacing, asymmetrical breasts, little or no breast changes in pregnancy or postpartum, and a need to begin supplementing their babies' nutrition within the first 2 weeks after giving birth. These respondents were most likely to actually have IGT. Because many in this sample were early in their breastfeeding experiences and still breastfeeding, our "long" breastfeeding duration was actually rather short: 4 months. However, we were still able to identify support factors that were received by those who continued breastfeeding versus those who weaned earlier. The most remarkable of these factors that emerged was whether a discussion of IGT by a health care provider affected breastfeeding duration. Among those whose postpartum breastfeeding support included information about IGT, more than 60% were still breastfeeding at or beyond 4 months; among those who did not receive postpartum information about IGT, fewer than one-fourth were still breastfeeding at the 4-month mark (p < .001).

Other findings from this analysis included the following:

- More mothers who perceived provider support for breastfeeding as "strong" breastfed for 4 months or more.

- When mothers perceived in-person or online help as effective, they were more likely to breastfeed longer.

- Mothers sought in-person help first but researched IGT more deeply online.

- Mothers who were instructed in milk expression, the use of an at-breast supplementing device, or the use of medications to increase milk output were more likely to breastfeed longer than mothers who did not receive these aspects of support.

It's obvious that information and specialized technical breast-feeding support are vital to the sustainability of breastfeeding for mothers with IGT. The mothers would agree, and I'll let them tell you how they feel. Their words may shock and upset you, as you may recall instances where, with the best intentions, you didn't tell a mother about a hunch you had or an observation you made. As breastfeeding supporters, it is our very job to trust the process of normal lactation, just as a homebirth midwife is expected to trust the process of normal birth! Yet, it is imperative that we begin to recognize the markers of potential abnormality, just as the midwife learns to recognize signs that the birth outcome will be better with a transfer away from home.

I feel like this is a political issue in that the breastfeeding commu-nity does not want to let out that some mothers can just not make enough milk. With such a simple check of even asking if a mom has had breast changes should be routine. I was so clueless that I was even happy that my breasts were not bigger since I didn't have the buy new bras!

The more I think about this, the more I feel that it is unethical for a health care provider to have information about my body and potential problems and withhold it from me. Especially a health-care provider who knows I am attending breastfeeding classes at her workplace and asking a million questions.

After seven or eight or nine months of prenatal appointments and care, your midwife; especially a midwife, should know your intentions. If I had a prenatal ultrasound and there was some potential problem detected in the fetus, and this problem was not disclosed because of how I may (or may not) react to this info there would be grounds for a lawsuit. Healthcare professionals have the obligation to inform and provide information. What we do with that information is our own choice. I was not given a choice.

Withholding information because I "may" decide to give up breastfeeding early isn't the health provider's call. I'm an intelligent woman and I appreciate being treated as such. I can only make an informed decision if I am informed. Some people might say, oh I'll formula feed then, and that's their choice based on that information. Some might say, thank goodness I know, I can read about this further and get prepared with drugs and herbs and having a decent breast pump. I didn't even have a pump when I had my daughter because I thought supply and demand would sort everything out.

One difficulty for me was that no one wanted to flat-out tell me that I had IGT...I was simply told "well, your breasts don't look normal for a breastfeeding woman" and "you might not have enough breast tissue to breastfeed." I didn't understand exactly what this meant or how definitive it was until following up with an Internet search. I held out hope that various things would improve my supply and none did—that has been pretty discouraging.

When my son was born 13 years ago, the lactation consultant came to our hospital room for a routine visit. I showed her my severely asymmetrical breasts and asked her point blank if she thought I would have any problems breastfeeding. She said emphatically no. It wasn't until my 3rd child was born two months ago that I learned of IGT and how it impacts my ability to breastfeed.

When We Know Better, We Do Better: Providing Support

It is extremely difficult physically and even more difficult emotionally. The encouragement and support are extremely important. It does feel good however to know that I'm not suffering alone.

Armed with information about the risk factors for lactation failure and insight into the experiences of mothers who have dealt with it, we may feel a growing sense of "knowing what we don't know" and have uncertainty about how to support a mother with IGT. Will she feel welcome and comfortable in your regular breastfeeding support group? Do you have the skills and information to help her choose and prepare an appropriate supplement for her baby? Few of us are trained psychologists or therapists. Who will these mothers turn to for the emotional support they need in mourning the loss of this aspect of mothering they so eagerly awaited?

It's amazing how information can empower you, even when it's not the news you were hoping to get. And it also shows how real emotional and practical support from professionals and other IGT women can lead to successful nursing.

The good news is that today's mothers have—and utilize— numerous support networks, thanks to social media platforms.

Karleen Gribble, Ph.D. (2001), offered a scholarly examination of these online "gathering places" in her article "Mother-to-Mother Support for Women Breastfeeding in Unusual Circumstances: A New Method for an Old Model." The Resource Chapter in this book presents several online places for mothers with IGT, which offer varying degrees of camaraderie and evidence. While there is no substitute for individualized clinical in-person support (even the best IBCLC can't assess milk transfer online!), the connection with other mothers who are experiencing the heartbreak of lactation failure is priceless and provides the motivation that they all need to keep breastfeeding as they are able.

Mothers with IGT who learn from other mothers' experiences will also likely come to you with new questions about potential therapies or solutions to their lactation issues. If you've read the other chapters in this book, you will be equipped to critically consider each idea or concept as it applies to that mother and her baby, and you'll be able to direct her to an informed, evidence-based choice about what to do next. That kind of empowerment permeates other areas of her mothering experience. The work you do to support the mother in setting and achieving *her* breastfeeding goals is vital and far-reaching.

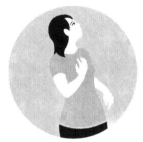

Chapter 8

Resources for More Information

There are lots of terrific resources in print and online that can help you "find sufficiency" in your breastfeeding experience. If you have IGT, there is a strong chance you are also insulin resistant. In Chapter 4, I offer a lot of information about insulin resistance and how it might affect your breastfeeding experience, but if you want to read some nonbreastfeeding commentary on this condition, this link offers some good information: *http://www. chiro.org/nutrition/ABSTRACTS/Insulin_Resistance.shtml.*

The Breastfeeding Mother's Guide to Making More Milk by Diana West and Lisa Marasco (2008) is really a prerequisite to this book because it addresses the many reasons a mother might struggle with low milk supply. If you haven't read it yet, be sure to get it—it may provide some additional pieces to your breastfeeding puzzle.

Internet Breastfeeding Support

In today's age of information, there are Internet "gathering places" for everything you can imagine, including breastfeeding and IGT. The IGT and Low Milk Supply Support Group is a closed Facebook group *(https://www.facebook.com/groups/IGTmamas/)* where members can post questions confidentially (only other members can see them, not your family or other Facebook friends) and provide unique, real-time support for each other in breastfeeding with IGT or low milk supply. There are comprehensive documents, which compile expert comments and guidance, photos of breasts for comparison, news of opportunities to participate in research, and a tightly moderated, friendly platform for getting and sharing information. You will need an admin's approval to join, but they usually approve requests within a day or two.

Perhaps the original online support "gathering place" for mothers with breastfeeding difficulties, MOBI Motherhood International (Mothers Overcoming Breastfeeding Issues; _http://www.mobimotherhood.org/)_, is still a clearinghouse of information and support:

The blog, *Diary of a Lactation Failure (http://diaryofalactationfailure. blogspot.com/)* by Nyssa Retter, IGT mom of four, offers great writing, resources, and a photo gallery for those wondering whether their breasts look like they are missing glandular tissue.

Not Everyone Can Breastfeed (http://noteveryonecanbreastfeed.com/pb/ wp_db0747f4/wp_db0747f4.html) is a website maintained by IGT mom, Heather Wong, that lists several resources for those in the early stages of information gathering.

Tongue Tie

It has been my clinical experience that most mothers who experience milk supply difficulties have a tongue tied or lip-tied baby. These mothers likely began their breastfeeding experiences with adequate glandular tissue and enough milk, but the baby's inability to properly remove milk and stimulate the production of more milk caused the mother's supply to dwindle over time.

It may be difficult to identify practitioners in your community who can identify and resolve tongue tie or lip tie, especially posterior tongue ties, which can be hard to see unless someone is very skilled. If you think that your baby may be tongue tied, print one or more of these resources and bring them to your IBCLC, pediatrician, pediatric dentist, or ear, nose, and throat (ENT) specialist. Check with your local breastfeeding support persons for suggestions of practitioners who might be skilled in repairing tongue and lip-ties.

Even if you've gotten this far in reading this book, tongue tie may still have been your breastfeeding problem. It is far, far more common than IGT. Tongue tie as a breastfeeding problem is becoming more understood by parents and the mainstream media, as this story illustrates: *http://www.wate.com/story/23060564/women-turn-to-dentist-office-to-solve-breastfeeding-issues.*

IBCLC Cathy Watson Genna's website *(http://www.cwgenna.com/quickhelp.html)* offers excellent pictures of posterior tongue ties and how to identify them.

Also see this resource, ideal for printing and taking to your pediatrician, IBCLC, or other health care provider: *http://www2.aap.org/breastfeeding/files/pdf/bbm-8-27%20Newsletter.pdf.*

Cathy Watson Genna's (2012) book, *Supporting Sucking Skills in Breastfeeding Infants* (2nd ed.), is a detailed, comprehensive resource for those dealing with complex issues of infant anatomy and feeding ability.

Pediatric dentist Dr. Larry Kotlow in Albany, New York, treats posterior tongue tie and lip tie with a dental laser. His website *(http://www.kiddsteeth.com/dental_topics.html#evaluate_and_diagnose_a_posterior_tongue_tie)* offers articles, photographs, and videos to help families and practitioners identify tongue ties that can affect breastfeeding.

Dr. Kotlow (2011) also published an article in *Clinical Lactation* (see the reference section) about how tongue tie can cause symptoms that mimic and are often mistaken for reflux in infants.

Alison Hazelbaker, Ph.D., IBCLC, has been serving breastfeeding families for years. Her tool for assessing tongue function and feeding capability is helpful for families and health care providers who want to understand why tongue tie is causing problems (Hazelbaker, 2010).

Help with Supplementation

Whether you choose to continue nursing your baby at your breasts, provide your milk for him, or both, you will need to choose and use an appropriate supplementation device to fit your unique situation.

An IBCLC can best help you learn how to incorporate the right tool into your feeding routine, so be sure to seek professional help after you've learned about your options from these resources.

Breastfeeding Without Birthing is a wonderful, heartfelt resource by Alyssa Schnell (2013), an IBCLC, who is also an adoptive mother. It offers sound, compassionate guidance for those who face unique breastfeeding challenges. Her chapter on supplementation methods is outstanding and definitely applicable to the IGT breastfeeding experience, as are many other sections of the book.

Another great book for families that choose to or need to combine breastfeeding with bottle-feeding is *Balancing Breast and Bottle: Reaching Your Breastfeeding Goals* by Amy Peterson, IBCLC, and

Mindy Harmer, SLP (2009). Written in easily understood language with lots of pictures, this resource offers solid guidance for choosing the feeding vessel that will be most compatible with your breasts and your baby's mouth. The bottle that works for one baby may not be the bottle that works best for yours. This book can help you cut through the marketing hype ("most like mom") and determine what teat shape and material will help your baby feed most effectively.

This article by Amber McCann, IBCLC, gives a good overview of at-breast supplementing tools and how to use them: _http://www.hygeiainc.com/digging-into-the-breastfeeding-tool-box-at-the-breast-supplementers/._

Figuring out how much your baby is getting and how much you need to supplement with can be confusing, especially when you're afraid to trust your body and your baby's cues. KellyMom (Kelly Bonyata, IBCLC) to the rescue! She offers an objective calculator to help you determine whether your baby is getting enough to eat so that you don't overfeed the supplement: _http://kellymom.com/bf/pumpingmoms/pumping/milkcalc/._

KellyMom also offers a wide selection of instructional articles for all things supplementing and alternative feeding, including some of my favorite resources for teaching healthy, appropriate bottle-feeding techniques (hint: a reclined baby with a bottle being dumped into his mouth is not a happy baby!). This link is to a handout you can print and bring to your baby's caregiver if you won't be doing all of the bottle-feeding yourself: _http://www.kellymom.com/store/freehandouts/bottle_feeding.pdf._

At KellyMom, you'll also find answers to questions about supplementing that you didn't even know you had, including a link to my favorite instructional piece on paced bottle-feeding by Dee Kassing, IBCLC: *http://kellymom.com/bf/pumpingmoms/feeding-tools/alternative-feeding/*.

It is both possible and preferable to "bottle-nurse" your bottle-fed baby by closely mimicking the posture, closeness, and connection of feeding at your breasts. The United Kingdom's, "Analytical Armadillo," Charlotte Young, IBCLC, offers this gem for techniques to bottle-feed with love and respect: *http://www.analyticalarmadillo.co.uk/2010/10/boosting-bottle-feeding-bonding-5-top.html.*

One of my favorite voices in the lactation support community is that of Diane Wiessinger, MS, IBCLC. Her words about breastfeeding and human nurturing are gentle, truthful, and supportive no matter where you are on your finding sufficiency journey. Her piece, "Staying in Touch" *(http://www.normalfed.com/Why/staytouch.html)* emphasizes the importance of staying physically close to your baby, especially if you are no longer breastfeeding him. She begins:

> If you and your baby are still struggling to make nursing work, if you stopped nursing before you wanted, or if you never really got started, first of all give yourself a big, warm hug for your efforts. With even a little breastmilk, or even a little nursing, you have given your baby an irreplaceable start on life. You can build on that wonderful start no matter how you feed your baby, if you remember that your baby's needs and expectations are still the same...

Lowmilksupply.org is owned and maintained by the authors of *The Breastfeeding Mother's Guide to Making More Milk,* so you can be assured that this information about when, how, and why to supplement is complete, easy to understand, and based on the vast knowledge of two of lactation's most experienced practitioners, Diana West and Lisa Marasco: *http://www.lowmilksupply.org/supplementing.shtml.*

The Academy of Breastfeeding Medicine (2009), in its Clinical Protocol #3: *Hospital Guidelines for the Use of Supplementary Feedings in the Healthy Term Breastfed Neonate,* explains the hows and whys (and, more importantly, the why nots) of offering supplemental feedings to the newborn baby still in the hospital. Most IGT moms will not need to supplement while still in the hospital. This is a great resource to print out and take with you if you're worried about hospital practices undermining your efforts to get breastfeeding off to the best start: *http://www.bfmed.org/Media/Files/Protocols/Protocol%20 3%20English%20Supplementation.pdf*

Even if supplementation is started in the first week of your baby's life, it's important to remember that his stomach is still so very tiny and can't hold a full bottle. He needs to be fed very small amounts, very frequently. This excellent visual illustration by Nancy Mohrbacher, IBCLC, of a newborn's growing stomach capacity in his first 10 days is another resource that you might consider taking with you to the hospital so you can protect your baby's early feeding experience and keep it as close to normal as is possible: *http://www.ameda.com. au/breastfeeding/breastfeeding-benefits/your-newborns-stomach-day-110.html.*

It's important to remember that our number one concern is feeding our babies, no matter how that needs to happen. There are good reasons to make bottle-feeding as much like breastfeeding as possible, no matter what's in the bottle, and this Native Mothering article offers excellent guidance on that topic: _http://nativemothering. com/2012/04/are-there-differences-between-breastfeeding-directly-and-bottle-feeding-expressed-milk/._

Infant feeding is a big part of what the USDA's Special Supplemental Nutrition Program for Women, Infants, and Children (WIC) takes care of. Their resources on bottle-feeding _(http://wicworks.nal.usda.gov/infants/ bottle-feeding)_ and on feeding a breastmilk substitute _(http://www.nal. usda.gov/wicworks/Topics/FG/Chapter4_InfantFormulaFeeding.pdf)_ are worth a read.

Choosing a Breastmilk Substitute

When you're mourning the loss of the exclusive breastfeeding relationship you hoped to share with your baby, the last thing you want to worry about is which breastmilk substitute is going to be the best one for your unique situation.

The unethical, predatory marketing practices and claims of the breastmilk-substitute industry only complicate an already overwhelming landscape of options. These links offer the facts without any hype.

There is a good commentary on organic breastmilk substitutes at: _http://foodbabe.com/2013/05/28/how-to-find-the-safest-organic-infant-formula/#more-13333._

If your baby doesn't seem to be well, what he's being fed may be to blame. The Academy of Breastfeeding Medicine (2011b) offers its ABM Clinical Protocol #24: *Allergic Proctocolitis in the Exclusively Breastfed Infant*. It explains why some babies who are exclusively breastfed or breastmilk-fed may experience colic, rashes, or rectal bleeding. This is an outstanding resource to print and bring to your child's health care provider if you have concerns about whether your baby's diet is being well-tolerated: *http://www.bfmed.org/Media/ Files/Protocols/Protocol24_English_120211.pdf*

Additional resources about fussy babies, bloody stools, and other symptoms that may be caused by dietary proteins (either via breastmilk or substitute) can be found at this website devoted completely to this topic: *http://infantproctocolitis.org/resources/.*

The facts about hydrolysate and amino-acid-based breastmilk substitutes can be found at this site. Yes, it is an industry site, but the information is presented in an unbiased manner: *http://www. neocate.com/blog/hydrolysate-formulas-vs-amino-acid-based-formulas/.*

The American Academy of Pediatrics (AAP) offers its guidance about hypoallergenic breastmilk substitutes at this site: *http://pediatrics. aappublications.org/content/106/2/346.full.*

If you're considering using a soy-based breastmilk substitute, there is some good information here about them: *http://www.askdrsears. com/topics/feeding-infants-toddlers/bottle-feeding/soy-formulas.*

The U.S. Food and Drug Administration (FDA) is responsible for ensuring that all products sold as infant nutrition products meet specific criteria. Those criteria and the products that the U.S. FDA regulates can be found here: _http://www.fda.gov/Food/GuidanceRegulation/ GuidanceDocumentsRegulatoryInformation/InfantFormula/ucm106456.htm._

Donor Milk

The practice of feeding human milk to human babies, even when breastfeeding is not possible, is not a "new thing." But for those of us born after the advent of commercially prepared breastmilk substitutes, our perceptions about how we feed our babies may be skewed by cultural practice and the marketing tactics of those who make a profit when babies are not fed human milk.

Be sure to read Chapter 5 before making a decision about obtaining and using donor milk, either from a milk bank or from a mother in your community.

The following essay frames the contemporary use of donor human milk in the United States: _http://thestir.cafemom.com/baby/143072/ more_moms_saying_no_to._

The following article explains how donor milk is processed by a Human Milk Banking Association of North America (HMBANA) milk bank: _https://www.hmbana.org/processing._

The largest Internet-based milk-sharing organization, Human Milk 4 Human Babies (HM4HB), offers a comprehensive resource for families as they consider the risks and benefits of obtaining and using human donor milk to feed their babies. This fact sheet is really required reading for anyone considering the use of donor milk that does not come from a milk bank: *http://hm4hb.net/faq/.*

Families and professionals will gain comfort and understanding from the blog post, *Supporting Families in Milk Sharing as an International Board Certified Lactation Consultant,* by Amber McCann (2012), IBCLC: *http://www.ambermccann.com/blog/milksharing.*

No matter what you decide to feed your baby, there may be people in your life who have issues with your choice. The article *Responding to Criticism,* by Marianne Vakiener (1999), offers some insight into dealing with those issues, whether they are held by people you love or others in your life: *http://www.lalecheleague.org/nb/nbjulaug99p116.html*

Medications and Breastfeeding

You may be worried that a medication you need is not compatible with breastfeeding because it's not safe for your baby to get through your milk.

More often, however, certain medications are not compatible with breastfeeding because they might lower your milk supply—and a mom with IGT doesn't need to add that to her list of worries.

These resources can help you and your health care providers determine what the best medicines are when you need them so that, in most cases, you can keep breastfeeding or producing milk for your baby.

The U.S. National Library of Medicine, part of the National Institutes of Health, produces this resource, accessible for free to anyone who needs it. It's also in app form if you want to keep it on your smartphone: _http://www.nlm.nih.gov/pubs/factsheets/lactmedfs.html._

The InfantRisk Center at the Texas Tech University Health Sciences Center, under the direction of Thomas Hale, Ph.D., offers a phone number you can call if you've got questions about a medication and whether it affects your ability to breastfeed. The InfantRisk Center also offers a textbook and other fee-based services, including a smartphone app and discussion forums at their website: _http://www.infantrisk.com/._

Antidepressant medication presents a common dilemma for breastfeeding mothers. This article offers a look at current research and guidance on this topic: _http://www.huffingtonpost.com/2014/04/15/breastfeeding-antidepressants_n_5144997.html._

Foods
You may be interested in trying particular foods to help boost your milk output.

Mother Food for Breastfeeding Mothers, by Hilary Jacobson (2004), offers an in-depth, well-researched look at lactogenic foods. An excellent summary can be found at this link: _http://www.mobimotherhood.org/mm/article-diet.aspx._

Because research is showing us very clearly that insulin plays a major role in milk production, diets that bring insulin under control and promote insulin sensitivity are showing promise for improving breast changes in pregnancy, as well as milk output once the baby arrives. Many mothers are finding success with a paleo type of diet, which emphasizes the intake of vegetables and protein, with a small amount of carbohydrates and excludes dairy, soy, grains, legumes, or processed foods. Whole9's "Whole30" plan *(http://whole9life.com/)* can help regulate insulin sensitivity. Even if milk output is not dramatically improved, overall heath might be. Many who've stuck with it for the whole 30 days do see an increase in their milk output, perhaps after an initial dip in supply during the first 7–10 days.

More research is needed on the effect of this (or similar) diet on milk output, but case reports of its success are very promising. Mothers who have finished the 30-day plan report losing weight (often after struggling with other meal plans and approaches to weight loss) and reducing or eliminating other health complaints.

Galactagogues

Everyone wants the "magic bullet" that will make milk production effortless and build new breast tissue. Unfortunately, the evidence to support the use of galactagogue herbs is very limited; most of it is based on anecdote and clinical observation not randomized trials. What works for one mother might not work for another.

If you are already maximizing your overall health through a sensible diet, daily physical activity, and adequate sleep, an herbal galactagogue may be able to give your milk production a boost, even if just a little bit, if you match your particular breastfeeding obstacle with the herb that might overcome it. Be sure to let your health care provider know if you are taking anything over the counter or that you obtained some other way. There may be interactions with other drugs or vitamins that you need to take, and some herbs are not recommended for those with particular medical conditions (for example, fenugreek can make thyroid problems worse).

The Academy of Breastfeeding Medicine (2011a) offers guidance for the use of herbs and pharmaceutical products (drugs) for boosting milk output: _http://www.bfmed.org/Media/Files/Protocols/Protocol%209%20-%20English%201st%20Rev.%20Jan%202011.pdf_

Herbalist, nurse, lactation consultant, and La Leche League Leader Sheila Humphrey has been advising nursing women about the use of herbs for a variety of reasons (not just milk production) for many years. Her resource is informative, comprehensive, and easy to understand Humphrey, S. (2003). *The nursing mother's herbal.* Minneapolis: Fairview Press.

Domperidone is a popular, if controversial, drug that is used to augment milk production in mothers who are not able to make enough milk on their own. It works by allowing prolactin to stay in the bloodstream longer than normal so that the prolactin receptors that are present (even if they are limited in number) have more time to take the prolactin up and use it. Be sure to carefully research all of the reasons that domperidone may or may not be a good option in your situation before you use it. This link offers general information but cannot serve as medical guidance about whether the side effects or risks of taking the medication will outweigh any increase in milk output that you may experience: _http://www.asklenore. info/breastfeeding/induced_lactation/domperidone_general.shtml._

Milk Expression

Part of your finding sufficiency journey may include expressing your milk in ways other than at your breast, by your baby. Pumping and hand-expressing your milk are both skills that require some practice and knowledge of your body. For an instructional video on how to effectively hand-express your milk, see Dr. Jane Morton's video at _http://newborns.stanford.edu/Breastfeeding/HandExpression.html._

See this video, also by Dr. Jane Morton, for some hands-on pumping instruction: _http://newborns.stanford.edu/Breastfeeding/MaxPro-duction.html._

For more information about choosing an efficient breast pump, including brand-specific suction and cycling ranges, see the _Breast-feeding in Combat Boots_ website link: _http://breastfeedingincombatboots. com/faq/pumping/choosing-breastpump/._

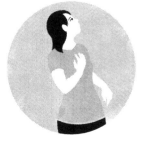 References

Academy of Breastfeeding Medicine. (2009). ABM clinical protocol #3: Hospital guidelines for the use of supplementary feedings in the healthy term breastfed neonate, revised 2009. *Breastfeeding Medicine,* 4, 175–182. Retrieved from http://www.bfmed.org/Media/Files/Protocols/Protocol%203%20English%20Supplementation.pdf

Academy of Breastfeeding Medicine. (2011a). ABM clinical protocol #9: Use of galactagogues in initiating or augmenting the rate of maternal milk secretion. *Breastfeeding Medicine,* 6, 41–46. Retrieved from http://www.bfmed.org/Media/Files/Protocols/Protocol%209%20-%20English%201st%20Rev.%20Jan%202011.pdf

Academy of Breastfeeding Medicine. (2011b). ABM clinical protocol #24: Allergic proctocolitis in the exclusively breastfed infant. *Breastfeeding Medicine,* 6, 435–440. Retrieved from http://www.bfmed.org/Media/Files/Protocols/Protocol24_English_120211.pdf

Akre, J. E., Gribble, K. D., & Minchin, M. (2011). Milk sharing: From private practice to public pursuit. *International Breastfeeding Journal,* 6, 8. doi: 10.1186/1746-4358-6-8

American Academy of Pediatrics, Section on Breastfeeding. (2012). Breastfeeding and the use of human milk. *Pediatrics,* 129, 2011–3552. doi: 10.1542/peds.2011-3552

Arbour, M. W., & Kessler, J. L. (2013). Mammary hypoplasia: Not every breast can produce sufficient milk. *Journal of Midwifery & Women's Health,* 58(4), 457-461. doi: 10.1111/jmwh.12070

Artini, P. G., DiBerardino, O. M., Papini, F., Genazzani, A. D., Simi, G., Ruggiero, M., & Cela, V. (2013). Endocrine and clinical effects of myo-inositol administration in policystyc ovary syndrome. A randomized study. *Gynecological Endocrinology,* 29, 375–379. Retrieved from http://www.ncbi.nlm.nih.gov/pubmed/23336594

Berlato, C., & Doppler, W. (2009). Selective response to insulin versus insulin-like growth factor-I and -II and up-regulation of insulin receptor splice variant B in the differentiated mouse mammary epithelium. *Endocrinology, 150,* 2924–2933. doi: 10.1210/en.2008-0668

Bodley, V., & Powers, D. (1999). Patient with insufficient glandular tissue experiences milk supply increase attributed to progesterone treatment for luteal phase defect. *Journal of Human Lactation, 15,* 339–343. doi: 10.1177/089033449901500415

Bonyata, K. (2011, October 28). *How much expressed milk will my baby need?* Retrieved from http://kellymom.com/bf/pumpingmoms/pumping/milkcalc/

Brannian, J. D., Zhao, Y., & McElroy, M. (1999). Leptin inhibits gonadotrophin-stimulated granulosa cell progesterone production by antagonizing insulin action. *Human Reproduction, 14,* 1445–1448. doi: 10.1093/humrep/14.6.1445

Brink, C. B., Viljoen, S. L., deKock, S. E., Stein, D. J., & Harvey, B. H. (2004). Effects of myo-inositol versus fluoxetine and imipramine pretreatments on serotonin 5HT2A and muscarinic acetylcholine receptors in human neuroblastoma cells. *Metabolic Brain Disease, 19*(1–2), 51–70.

Brody, J. (2014, April 15). A number that may not add up. *The New York Times.* Retrieved from http://well.blogs.nytimes.com/2014/04/14/a-number-that-may-not-add-up/

Burt Solorzano, C. M., & McCartney, C. R. (2010). *Obesity and the pubertal transition in boys and girls.* Reproduction, 140, 399–410. doi: 10.1530/REP-10-0119

Centers for Disease Control and Prevention. (2012). *Breastfeeding report card 2012, United States: Outcome indicators.* Retrieved from http://www.cdc.gov/breastfeeding/data/reportcard2.htm

Chantry, C. J., Nommsen-Rivers, L. A., Peerson, J. M., Cohen, R. J., & Dewey, K. G. (2011). Excess weight-loss in first-born breastfed newborns relates to maternal intrapartum fluid balance. *Pediatrics, 127*, e171–e179. doi: 10.1542/peds.2009-2663

Chapman, D., & Pérez-Escamilla, R. (1999). Identification of risk factors for delayed onset of lactation. *Journal of the American Dietetic Association, 99*, 450–454.

Codex Alimentarius Commission. (1981). *Standard for infant formula and formulas for special medical purposes intended for infants. Codex Stan 72-1981.* Retrieved from http://www.codexalimentarius.org/input/download/.../288/CXS_072e.pdf

de Carvalho, M., Robertson, S. Friedman, A., & Klaus, M. (1983). Effect of frequent breast-feeding on early milk production and infant weight gain. *Pediatrics, 72*, 307–311.

Dewey, K. G. (2001). Nutrition, growth, and complimentary feeding of the breastfed infant. *Pediatric Clinics of North America, 48*, 87–104.

Dykes, F., & Williams, C. (1999). Falling by the wayside: A phenomenological exploration of perceived breastmilk inadequacy in lactating women. *Midwifery, 15*, 232–246.

Ezzo, G., & Bucknam, R. (1995). *On becoming babywise.* Chatsworth, CA: Parent Wise Solutions.

Ezzo, G., & Ezzo, A. M. (1993). *Growing kids God's way.* Chatsworth, CA: Growing Families International Press.

Fenton, S. E., Hamm, J. T., Birnbaum, L. S., & Youngblood, G. L. (2002). Persistent abnormalities in the rat mammary gland following gestational and lactational exposure to 2,3,7,8-tetrachlorodibenzo-p-dioxin (TCDD). *Toxicological Sciences, 67*, 63–74.

Fife, S., Gill, P., Hopkins, M., Angello, C., Boswell, S., & Nelson, K. M. (2011). Metoclopramide to augment lactation, does it work? A randomized trial. *Journal of Maternal-Fetal and Neonatal Medicine, 24,* 1317–1320. doi: 10.3109/14767058.2010.549255

Flegal, K. M., Carroll, M. D., Kit, B. K., & Ogden, C. L. (2012). Prevalence of obesity and trends in the distribution of body mass index among U.S. adults, 1999–2010. *Journal of the American Medical Association, 307,* 491–497. Retrieved from *http://jama.jamanetwork.com/article.aspx?articleid=1104933*

Forinash, A. B., Yancey, A. M., Barnes, K. N., & Myles, T. D. (2012). The use of galactagogues in the breastfeeding mother. *Annals of Pharmacotherapy, 46,* 1392–1404. doi: 10.1345/aph.1R167

Genna, C. W. (2012). *Supporting sucking skills in breastfeeding infants* (2nd ed.). Sudbury, MA: Jones & Bartlett.

Gerli, S., Papaleo, E., Ferrari, A., & DiRenzo, G. C. (2007). Randomized, double blind placebo-controlled trial: Effects of myo-inositol on ovarian function and metabolic factors in women with PCOS. *European Review for Medical and Pharmacological Sciences, 11,* 347–354.

Gladen, B. C., & Rogan, W. J. (1995). DDE and shortened duration of lactation in a northern Mexican town. *American Journal of Public Health, 85,* 504–508.

Goldman, A. S., Goldblum, R. M., & Garza, C. (1983). Immunologic components of human milk during the second year of lactation. *Acta Paediatrica Scandinavica, 72,* 461–462.

Gribble, K. D. (2001). Mother-to-mother support for women breastfeeding in unusual circumstances: A new method for an old model. *Breastfeeding Review, 9*(3), 13–19.

Gribble, K. D., & Hausman, B. L. (2012). Milk sharing and formula feeding: Infant feeding risks in comparative perspective? *Australasian Medical Journal, 5,* 275–283. doi: 10.4066/AMJ.2012.1222

Guillette, E. A., Conard, C., Lares, F., Aguilar, M. G., McLachlan, J.,

& Guillette, L. J., Jr. (2006). Altered breast development in young girls from an agricultural environment. *Environmental Health Perspectives, 114,* 471–475.

Hale, T. W. (2012). *Medications and Mother's Milk 2012: A Manual of Lactational Pharmacology.* Plano, TX: Hale Publishing.

Hari, V. (2013). *How to find the safest organic infant formula.* Retrieved from *http://foodbabe.com/2013/05/28/how-to-find-the-safest-organic-infant-formula/*

Hazelbaker, A. K. (2010). *Tongue tie: Morphogenesis, impact, assessment, and treatment.* Columbus, OH: Aidan and Eva Press.

Hilgers, T. W. (2006). *The medical & surgical practice of NaPro technology.* Omaha, NE: Pope Paul VI Institute.

Hue-Beauvais, C., Chavatte-Palmer, P., Aujean, E., Dahirel, M., Laigre, P., Pechoux, C.,…Charlier, M. (2011). An obesogenic diet started before puberty leads to abnormal mammary gland development during pregnancy in the rabbit. *Developmental Dynamics, 240,* 347–356.

Huggins, K. E., Petok, E. S., & Mireles, O. (2000). Markers of lactation insufficiency: A study of 34 mothers. *Current issues in clinical lactation* (pp. 25–35). Sudbury, MA: Jones & Bartlett.

Human Milk 4 Human Babies Global Network. (n.d.). Frequently asked questions. Retrieved from *http://hm4hb.net/faq/*

Humphrey, S. (2003). *The nursing mother's herbal.* Minneapolis: Fairview Press.

Ingram, J., Taylor, H., Churchill, C., Pike, A., & Greenwood, R. (2012) Metoclopramide or domperidone for increasing maternal breast-milk output: A randomized controlled trial. *Archives of Disease in Childhood: Fetal and Neonatal Edition, 97,* F241–F245. doi: 10.1136/archdischild-2011-300601

Jacobson, H. (2004). *Mother food for breastfeeding mothers.* Rosalind Press.

Jones, E., Dimmock, P. W., & Spencer, S. A. (2001). A randomised controlled trial to compare methods of milk expression after preterm delivery. *Archives of Disease in Childhood: Fetal and Neonatal Edition,* 85, F91–F95.

Kasai, A., Hiramatsu, N., Hayakawa, K., Yao, J., Maeda, S., & Kitamura, M. (2006). High levels of dioxin-like potential in cigarette smoke evidenced by *in vitro* and *in vivo* biosensing. *Cancer Research,* 66, 7143–7150. doi: 10.1158/0008-5472.CAN-05-4541

Keim, S. A., Hogan, J. S., McNamara, K. A., Gudimetta, V., Dillon C. E., Kwiek, J. J., & Geraghty, S. R. (2013). Microbial contamination of human milk purchased via the Internet. *Pediatrics,* 32, e1227–e1235. doi: 10.1542/peds.2013-1687

Kotlow, L. (2011). Infant reflux and aerophagia associated with the maxillary lip-tie and ankyloglossia (tongue tie). *Clinical Lactation,* 2–4, 25–29. Retrieved from *http://kiddsteeth.com/articles/aerophagia_2011.pdf*

Lawrence, R. A., & Lawrence, R. M. (2011). *Breastfeeding: A guide for the medical profession* (7th ed.). Maryland Heights, MO: Elsevier Mosby.

Lemay, D. G., Ballard, O. A., Hughes, M. A., Morrow, A. L., Horseman, N. D., & Nommsen-Rivers, L. A. (2013). RNA sequencing of the human milk fat layer transcriptome reveals distinct gene expression profiles at three stages of lactation. *PLoS One,* 8, e67531. doi: 10.1371/journal.pone.0067531

Lyford, E. (2003). *How to bottle-feed the breastfed baby: Tips for a breastfeeding supportive style of bottle-feeding.* Retrieved from *http://www.kellymom.com/store/freehandouts/bottle_feeding.pdf*

Macias, H., & Hinck, L. (2012). Mammary gland development. *Wiley Interdisciplinary Reviews. Developmental Biology,* 1, 533–557. doi: 10.1002/wdev.35

Marasco, L., Marmet, C., & Shell, E. (2000). Polycystic ovarian syndrome: A connection to insufficient milk supply? *Journal of Human Lactation, 16,* 143–148.

Markey, C. M., Rubin, B. S., Soto, A. M., & Sonnenschein, C. (2003). Endocrine disruptors: From Wingspread to environmental developmental biology. *Journal of Steroid Biochemical Molecular Biology,* 83(1–5), 235–244.

Matsuno, A. Y., Esrey, K. L., Perrault, H., & Koski, K. G. (1999). Low intensity exercise and varying proportions of dietary glucose and fat modify milk and mammary gland compositions and pup growth. *Journal of Nutrition, 129,* 1167–1175

McAuley, K. A., Williams, S. M., Mann, J. I., Walker, R. J., Lewis-Barned, P. J., Temple, L. A., & Duncan, A. W. (2001). Diagnosing insulin resistance in the general population. *Diabetes Care, 24,* 460–464. Retrieved from *http://care.diabetesjournals.org/content/24/3/460.full#T3*

McCann, A. D. (2012, September 21). Supporting families in milk sharing as an International Board Certified Lactation Consultant. Retrieved from *http://ambermccann.com/milksharing/*

McMeekin, S., Jansen, E., Mallan, K., Nicholson, J., Magarey, A., & Daniels, L. (2013). Associations between infant temperament and early feeding practices: A cross-sectional study of Australian mother–infant dyads from the NOURISH randomised controlled trial. *Appetite, 60,* 239–245. doi: 10.1016/j.appet.2012.10.005

Mohammad, M. A., Sunehag, A. L., & Haymond, M. W. (2009). Effect of dietary macronutrient composition under moderate hypocaloric intake on maternal adaptation during lactation. *American Journal of Clinical Nutrition, 89,* 1821–1827. doi: 10.3945/ajcn.2008.26877

Moore, G. S. (2007). *Living with the Earth: Concepts in environmental health science* (pp. 201–204). Boca Raton, FL: Taylor & Francis.

Mortel, M., & Mehta, S. D. (2013). Systematic review of the efficacy of herbal galactagogues. *Journal of Human Lactation, 29,* 154–162. doi: 10.1177/0890334413477243

Morton, J. A. (1994). The clinical usefulness of breastmilk sodium in the assessment of lactogenesis. *Pediatrics, 93,* 802–806.

Neifert, M. R., & Bunik, M. (2013). Overcoming clinical barriers to exclusive breastfeeding. *Pediatric Clinics of North America, 60,* 115–145. doi: 10.1016/j.pcl.2012.10.001

Newman, J., & Kernerman, E. (2009). *Starting solid foods.* Retrieved from *http://www.breastfeedinginc.ca/content.php?pagename=doc-SSF*

Noel-Weiss, J., Woodend, A. K., Peterson, W. E., Gibb, W., & Groll, D. L. (2011). An observational study of associations among maternal fluids during parturition, neonatal output, and breastfed newborn weight loss. *International Breastfeeding Journal, 6,* 9. doi: 10.1186/1746-4358-6-9

Nommsen-Rivers, L. A., Chantry, C. J., Peerson, J. M., Cohen, R. J., & Dewey, K. G. (2010). Delayed onset of lactogenesis among first-time mothers is related to obesity and factors associated with ineffective breastfeeding. *American Journal of Clinical Nutrition, 92,* 574–584. doi: 10.3945/ajcn.2010.29192

Odom, E. C., Li, R., Scanlon, K. S., Perrine, C. G., & Grummer-Strawn, L. (2013). Reasons for earlier than desired cessation of breastfeeding. Pediatrics, 131, e726–e732. doi: 10.1542/peds.2012-1295

Ogden, C. L., Carroll, M. D., Kit, B. K., & Flegal, K. M. (2012). Prevalence of obesity and trends in body mass index among U.S. children and adolescents, 1999–2010. *Journal of the American Medical Association, 307,* 483–490. Retrieved from *http://jama.jamanetwork.com/Mobile/article.aspx?articleid=1104932*

Ostrum, K. M., & Ferris, A. M. (1993). Prolactin concentrations in serum and milk of mothers with and without insulin-dependent diabetes mellitus. *American Journal of Clinical Nutrition, 58*, 49–53.

Parry, K., Taylor, E., Hall-Dardess, P., Walker, M., & Labbok, M. (2013). Understanding women's perceptions of infant formula advertising. *Birth, 40*, 115–124. doi: 10.1111/birt.12044.

Peterson, A., & Harmer, M. (2009). *Balancing breast and bottle: Reaching your breastfeeding goals.* Amarillo, TX: Hale Publishing.

Ramsay, D. T., Kent, J. C., Hartmann, R. A., & Hartmann, P. E. (2005). Anatomy of the lactating breast refined with ultrasound imaging. *Journal of Anatomy, 206*(6), 525-534. doi: 10.1111/j.1469-7580.2005.00417.x

Rasmussen, K. M., Hilson, J. A., & Kjolhede, C. L. (2001). Obesity may impair lactogenesis II. *Journal of Nutrition, 131*, 3009S–3011S.

Rasmussen, K. M., & Kjolhede, C. L. (2004). Prepregnant overweight and obesity diminish the prolactin response to suckling in the first week postpartum. *Pediatrics, 113*, 3465–3471.

Riordan, J., & Wambach, K. (2010). Breastfeeding and human lactation (4th ed.). Sudbury, MA: Jones & Bartlett.

Roche-Paull, R. (2012). *Choosing a breastpump.* Retrieved from *http://www.breastfeedingincombatboots.com/faq/pumping/choosing-breastpump/*

Rudel, R. A., Fenton, S. E., Ackerman, J. M., Euling, S. Y., & Makris, S. L. (2011). Environmental exposures and mammary gland development: State of the science, public health implications, and research recommendations. *Environmental Health Perspectives, 119*, 1053–1061. doi: 10.1289/ehp.1002864

Schnell, A. (2013). *Breastfeeding without birthing: A breastfeeding guide for mothers through adoption, surrogacy, and other special circumstances.* Amarillo, TX: Praeclarus Press.

Sears, W. (2013). *Soy formulas?* Retrieved from http://www.askdrsears.com/topics/feeding-infants-toddlers/bottle-feeding/soy-formulas

Slusser, W., & Frantz, K. (2001). High-technology breastfeeding. *Pediatric Clinics of North America, 48,* 505–516.

Sun, Z., Shushanov, S., LeRoith, D., & Wood, T. L. (2011). Decreased IGF type 1 receptor signaling in mammary epithelium during pregnancy leads to reduced proliferation, alveolar differentiation, and expression of insulin receptor substrate (IRS)-1 and IRS-2. *Endocrinology, 152,* 3233–3245. doi: 10.1210/en.2010-1296

Thorley, V. (2005). Breast hypoplasia and breastfeeding: A case history. *Breastfeeding Review, 13*(2), 13-16.

U.S. Department of Agriculture. (2004). *Chapter 4: Infant formula feeding.* WIC Works Resource System. Retrieved from http://www.nal.usda.gov/wicworks/Topics/FG/Chapter4_InfantFormulaFeeding.pdf

U.S. Department of Agriculture, Food and Nutrition Service. (2013). *Frequently asked questions about WIC.* Retrieved from http://www.fns.usda.gov/wic/frequently-asked-questions-about-wic

U.S. Department of Health and Human Services, Healthy People 2020 (2012, October 30). *Maternal, infant, and child health: Objectives.* Retrieved from http://www.healthypeople.gov/2020/topicsobjectives2020/objectiveslist.aspx?topicid=26

U.S. Department of Health and Human Services, National Institutes of Health. (2013, January 23). *Panel recommends changing name of common disorder in women.* Retrieved from http://www.nih.gov/news/health/jan2013/od-23.htm

U. S. Environmental Protection Agency. (2011). *Persistent bioaccumulative and toxic (PBT) chemical program: Dioxins and furans.* Retrieved from http://www.epa.gov/pbt/pubs/dioxins.htm

Vakiener, M. (1999). Responding to criticism. *New Beginnings, 16*(4),

116–119. Retrieved from *http://www.lalecheleague.org/nb/nbju-laug99p116.html*

Vanky, E., Nordskar, J. J., Leithe, H., Hjorth-Hansen, A. K., Marti-nussen, M., & Carlsen, S. M. (2012). Breast size increment during pregnancy and breastfeeding in mothers with polycystic ovarian syndrome: A follow-up study of a randomized controlled trial on metformin versus placebo. *BJOG: An International Journal of Obstetrics and Gynaecology, 119,* 1403–1409. doi: 10.1111/j.1471-0528.2012.03449.x

von Wartburg, L. (2007). *What's a glucose clamp, anyway?* Retrieved from *http://www.diabeteshealth.com/read/2007/11/06/5500/whats-a-glucose-clamp-anyway/*

Vorderstrasse, B. A., Fenton, S. E., Bohn, A. A., Cundiff, J. A., & Lawrence, B. P. (2004). A novel effect of dioxin: Exposure during pregnancy severely impairs mammary gland differentiation. *Toxicological Sciences, 78,* 248–257.

Wada, T., Hori, S., Sugiyama, M., Fujisawa, E., Nakano, T., Tsunecki, H.,...Sasaoka, T. (2010). Progesterone inhibits glucose uptake by affecting diverse steps of insulin signaling in 3T3-L1 adipocytes. *American Journal of Physiology, Endocrinology, and Metabolism, 298,* E881–E888. doi: 10.1152/ajpendo.00649.2009

Wagner, U., Handke, L., Dörfel, D., & Walter, H. (2012). An experimental decision-making paradigm to distinguish guilt and regret and their self-regulating function via loss averse choice behavior. *Frontiers in Psychology, 3,* 431. doi: 10.3389/fpsyg.2012.00431

Walker, M. (n.d.). *"Just one bottle won't hurt"—or will it?* Retrieved from *http://www.health-e-learning.com/articles/JustOneBottle.pdf*

Watkins, S., Meltzer-Brody, S., Zolnoun, D., & Stuebe, A. (2011). Early breastfeeding experiences and postpartum depression.

Journal of Obstetrics and Gynecology, 118, 214–221. doi: 10.1097/ AOG.0b013e3182260a2d

Weschler, T. (2006). *Taking charge of your fertility: 10th anniversary edition.* New York: HarperCollins.

West, D., & Marasco, L. (2008). *The breastfeeding mother's guide to making more milk.* New York: McGraw-Hill.

World Health Organization. (1981). *International code of marketing of breastmilk substitutes.* Retrieved from *http://www.who.int/nutrition/ publications/code_english.pdf*

World Health Organization. (2003). *Global strategy for infant and young child feeding.* Retrieved from http://www.who.int/nutrition/publications/gs_infant_feeding_text_eng.pdf

Young, C. (2010). *Boosting bottle-feeding bonding—5 top tips.* Retrieved from *http://www.analyticalarmadillo.co.uk/2010/10/boosting-bottle-feeding-bonding-5-top.html*

Zapantis, A., Steinberg, J. G., & Schilit, L. (2012). Use of herbals as galactagogues. *Journal of Pharmacy Practice,* 25, 222–231. doi: 10.1177/0897190011431636

Zoppou, C., Barry, S. I., & Mercer, G. N. (1997). Comparing breastfeeding and breast pumps using a computer model. *Journal of Human Lactation,* 13, 195–202. doi: 10.1177/089033449701300307

30541936R00129

Made in the USA
San Bernardino, CA
16 February 2016